THE .... RE

HANDBOOK FOR NEVADA

The ESSENTIAL ELDERCARE HANDBOOK *for* NEVADA

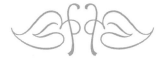

Kim Boyer, JD
and
Mary Shapiro, MSG, CMC

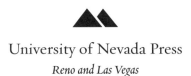

University of Nevada Press
Reno and Las Vegas

The information in this book does not offer and should not
be construed as providing legal, accounting, or tax advice or
professional services.

University of Nevada Press, Reno, Nevada 89557 USA
Copyright © 2014 by University of Nevada Press
All rights reserved
Manufactured in the United States of America
Design by Kathleen Szawiola

Library of Congress Cataloging-in-Publication Data
Boyer, Kim, 1965–
The essential eldercare handbook for Nevada / Kim Boyer, JD and
Mary Shapiro, MSG, CMC.
pages cm
Includes index.
ISBN 978-0-87417-941-5 (pbk. : alk. paper) —
ISBN 978-0-87417-942-2 (e-book)
1. Older people—Care—Nevada. 2. Caregivers—Nevada.
3. Long-term care facilities—Nevada 4. Estate planning—Nevada.
I. Shapiro, Mary, 1949– II. Title.
HV1468.N3B69 2014
362.609793—dc23   2013039749

The paper used in this book meets the requirements of American
National Standard for Information Sciences—Permanence of Paper
for Printed Library Materials, ANSI/NISO Z39.48-1992 (R2002).
Binding materials were selected for strength and durability.

First Printing
22   21   20   19   18   17   16   15   14
5   4   3   2   1

MARY

To my beloved and beautiful sister, Cornelia, who taught me
the meaning of loyalty, love, and laughter, and to her children,
Maryalyce and Regina, who inspire me every day.

KIM

To Mom, I love you with my whole heart.

AND TOGETHER,

we dedicate this book to caregivers who live and love
with courage and compassion.

CONTENTS

We all struggle to keep control over our lives and to maintain our balance. If you or your loved one is facing an illness, you are beginning to realize what a loss of control can do to your life. Caring for a loved one can put a strain on your family time, your employment time, and your plans for your own retirement. Caring for a spouse can put you under tremendous stress, combined with worry about loss of control over your financial security.

This book is designed to give you knowledge about and options for caregiving and protecting your financial security, specifically for those in Nevada. In our many years of helping families in Nevada, we have seen that people are often confused or unsure of what to do. Some even have wrong information. Our goal is to tell you in simple language not just what the problem is, but what you can do about it.

We start by helping you understand the aging process and when and if you need to intervene in your loved one's life. This is a tricky issue with many pros and cons. We clarify this subject matter and discuss some of those red lights that signal problems needing your intervention. We discuss balancing your life plans with the possibility of becoming a caregiver and provide tips and techniques for common caregiver issues.

Care is expensive. Without careful planning, a catastrophic illness can wipe out the life savings of most families. We explain in plain English what the Nevada rules are and how you can preserve assets and attain peace of mind. This book can educate you on the basic concepts of Nevada Medicaid, as well as more advanced asset-protection techniques. We cover the income limits and asset limits for Nevada Medicaid and explain what you can do under Nevada law to protect your assets. We also discuss what you cannot do.

This book also explains veterans' benefits for long-term care. There is a great benefit for veterans or surviving spouses who qualify that will give a monthly allowance even if the veteran does not have a service-connected disability. We also discuss estate planning, financial planning, health care planning, and the Affordable Care Act. We include a resource directory, with detailed resources available in Nevada.

This book combines the professional experience of an elder law attorney and a geriatric care manager. After reading this book, you can make your decisions, however difficult they may be, with the confidence that you are acting in an informed and responsible manner. We hope this leads you to successful and positive solutions.

ACKNOWLEDGMENTS

We gratefully thank many people for their inspiration and help in writing this book.

We thank Charles Bernick, MD, neurologist, associate medical director at the Cleveland Clinic Lou Ruvo Center for Brain Health, Las Vegas, for sharing his time and expertise with us. We also thank Kenneth J. Doka, PhD, MDIV, professor of gerontology at the graduate school of the College of New Rochelle; Lutheran minister; senior consultant to the Hospice Foundation of America; and editor of HFA's *Living with Grief* book series, its *Journeys* newsletter, and numerous other books and publications, who has long been a mentor to Mary.

We thank Phyllis Militello, MPA, former assistant director at Nevada Geriatric Education Center. Matt Becker, senior acquisitions editor at the University of Nevada Press, has been a joy to work with. His guidance and good counsel helped see this book through to its completion and publication. Our editor, Melanie Mallon, provided invaluable advice and guidance. Many thanks to Benjamin Drown, Joyce Brozovich, Laura Gover, Matthew and Gregory Valko, Caitlyn Drown, Holly Jeffries, Luisa Heizer, and Catherine Marquez for their continuous patience, encouragement, and excellent comments as we wrote and revised our manuscript.

We acknowledge our families, friends, and the entire team at Boyer Law Group for being motivators and cheerleaders whenever we stressed about the book. We could not have done it without you. Most of all, we could not have written this without all the families who have honored us by sharing their concerns, confusion, and joy as they journeyed through the aging and caregiving process.

THE ESSENTIAL ELDERCARE
HANDBOOK FOR NEVADA

CHAPTER ONE

An Eldercare Overview

The Growing Need for Eldercare

Patricia and Jim Peterson live in Las Vegas and have been married for thirty years. They are looking forward to retirement in the not-too-distant future. Jim will be sixty-two on his last day of work. He will exit the world of work with social security, a fairly decent pension, carefully acquired assets, and good health.

He will not miss getting up at the crack of dawn to commute or the pressure of time clocks, deadlines, and office politics. Patricia is fifty-three. She was a stay-at-home mom who cared for three children, all with families of their own. One is newly divorced with two children and not much money.

The Petersons want to buy an RV and tour the United States, visiting spots they have talked about for years and seeing friends. Jim is an avid fisherman, and he and Patricia are talking about buying a small boat they can hook up to the RV. What Patricia and Jim do not talk about, however, is how they will address the aging of their parents.

Patricia's mom and dad are in their early eighties and live over two thousand miles away, in Philadelphia, Pennsylvania. Patricia speaks with them by phone about once a week, and they see each other once a year.

Jim's dad is a widower, retired and living on his own in Reno, Nevada. He is a feisty ninety-two and tells Jim he is doing "just fine," although Jim is getting concerned. Dad has had a few fender benders, and it is getting harder to hold a telephone conversation that makes much sense anymore.

The Petersons have no real idea of their parents' assets or needs. They have never broached the subject of what would or should happen if there were a medical crisis requiring intervention, and, of course, they have never even considered planning for their own aging needs. They do not see themselves as old, and it has never entered their minds to involve their own children in this discussion.

Maddy and Joe live in Henderson, Nevada. They are part of the healthiest, most educated, independent cohort in the United States, the post–World War II baby boomer generation, and proud of it. Although hit by the economic downturn, they feel fortunate.

Maddy's widowed mother, Lucy, lives alone in Elko, Nevada. She has arthritis, kidney problems, high blood pressure, and she recently had a fall. Lucy insists on staying at home. Her only income is social security and a small pension from her deceased husband. No one ever thought of long-term care insurance, nor made a plan of what Mom might need or want. It will cost thousands of dollars each month to keep her at home with help. Joe's stepmom, Liz, is also beginning to need more help, but his dad, Richard, is currently able to handle matters. Joe and Maddy's retirement plans are changing in a way they did not expect. They love their family and will not abandon them, yet they hate the position they are in. Resentment, fear, and guilt make logic disappear. There is nothing worse than feeling out of control and waiting for the next crisis to happen.

Approximately 78 million baby boomers are about to reach retirement age. In 2011, the first of these baby boomers began blowing out the candles on their sixty-fifth birthday cakes. Moreover, the eighty-plus group is the fastest-growing demographic segment in the United States. The number of people one hundred years and older has exploded as well. In Nevada, the elderly population grew by more than 70 percent between 1990 and 2000—the largest senior citizen population growth in the country. The population of Nevadans age sixty-five and over is expected to increase 264 percent between 2000 and 2030.

We are certainly fortunate to live in a society that has pushed the boundaries of life expectancy. Baby boomers, the seniors who remain fully employed, and the generation that preceded them, are facing the issues of their own successful aging, while dealing with the challenges of caring for at least one elderly family member, often many more than just one. It is not unusual to be asked to care for your parents, your in-laws, your spouse, and even an ex-husband or wife. The frightening reality is that retirement savings may be used up by eldercare services and precious time lost searching for services that may not even exist. We are a society that is living longer, but not always happier, lives.

People in their sixties or seventies commonly find themselves working, caring for their elderly family members, taking care of their own concerns, and sometimes being responsible for their children and grandchildren too.

The scary truth is that the newly retired person better have sufficient money set aside to support themselves and their aging relatives. But few do. For some, retirement will come only when they can no longer physically work. In a recent AARP survey, "Boomers at Midlife," 23 percent of boomers said the worst aspect of their life was personal finance, and only 58 percent believed they could meet their financial goals for retirement. A survey conducted by Merrill Lynch found that nearly 80 percent of boomers intend to keep working beyond age sixty-five.

Like a pebble thrown in the lake of aging challenges, the model of the working elderly only adds ripples to the dilemma of who will be available to take care of those loved ones needing help. How people plan and deal with aspects of their own aging and those they love will have a powerful influence on the culture and economy of the United States.

When the Time for Care Has Come

Aging should not be a scary time. It is a time when you are mature enough to make conscious decisions about how to maintain your power and stay in control. There now exists a unique opportunity to use life experience and leisure time to acquire new skills and achieve the highest possible level of successful aging. This is all contingent, however, on planning.

Childhood, adolescence, youth, and middle age—all the important markers of life—need preparation and monitoring for success. Aging into elderhood is no different in that respect. Your adult children may very well be the ones reluctant to discuss topics such as what you want them to do if you become unable to make health decisions or what your end-of-life wishes are.

They may tell you, "Oh, Mom, you and Dad will live forever. We don't need to have this conversation." They do not want to face the possibility that you may someday require their assistance. They want you to stay young and healthy and independent forever. To admit any other scenario will open up the likelihood of loss and grief and, yes, the changes to their lives that may occur if you become fragile and ill. It is easier to avoid the issues, but avoidance can mean a lost opportunity to plan ahead.

You need to make sure your loved ones understand how important it is for them and for the family to make a plan together as early as possible. When any important life decision is made without careful consideration, someone will inevitably say or think, "If only I had" or "I should have" or "If only I had known." Decisions that are made in haste are often the most regretted.

We do not want that to happen to you or your loved ones when dealing with aging issues. You need to know how to make the necessary and practical preparations to avoid as many crises as you can. You cannot control all the circumstances that life may throw at you or at your loved ones, but you can make sure you all have the information necessary to act with confidence, rather than react in a panic. With more knowledge, you can create a better plan.

Make a Plan

In our society, aging is like the proverbial elephant in the room. We flee from the word *old,* and multibillion-dollar industries and scams have used the fear of aging to launch antiaging products, magic potions, and cosmetic surgery. The promise is to extend our youth forever. We strive to stay fit, look good, and make the most of our bodies and minds. But we also need to put a dose of reality into the picture. You are fortunate if your loved ones initiate sitting down with important family members to outline what to do for them as their needs increase. It then becomes a matter of setting an agenda of topics, deciding what roles family members are able or willing to take in eldercare, and figuring out how to determine when to begin the caregiving process.

Your family may be able to create such a care plan on their own, or you might like to involve a neutral facilitator, who can move the process along and not allow it to get bogged down or off topic. We invite you to use our "Guide to the Family Meeting," in appendix A of this book, as a starting point for discussion.

If your loved ones are competent, you can voice your opinion, but they will determine what their future will look like. Do not let family dynamics ruin this exercise. You may think your brother is not the right one to act in a certain capacity. Is that because of a real concern or is it an issue between siblings? For example, your parents may overlook the eldest and put the baby in charge of finances. Do not allow hurt feelings to create a rift with your parents or siblings.

If your loved ones talk about alternative housing arrangements, but you cannot bear for them to leave the family home, you must be prepared to follow their wishes or decline the role of primary caregiver. Your loved one should be involved in decision making as much as possible. It does not work for the family to meet without the loved ones needing care and then tell them about the decisions made. We recommend a family meeting as soon as possible before a crisis arises. Often, however, it takes a sudden illness or a diagnosis of dementia before families begin to recognize the enormity of eldercare and come together to figure out what to do and who will do what. Again, we cannot emphasize enough: The sooner you plan, the better.

Patricia and Jim Peterson have a lot to look forward to as their journey into retirement begins. Let's talk a bit about the considerations they need to address to make a successful plan for their future.

What, Sell the Family Home?

The Petersons love their home. It is a big two-story, with nooks and crannies their children used for hiding places. Patricia has a vegetable garden that feeds not only the neighbors but the rabbits and birds as well. The house has been a financial lifesaver more than once, with second mortgages used for college tuition and an unexpected job loss. The children love it and consider it the family home.

A home is a financial asset, and it is an emotional connection to family and friends. Here are some questions you need to ask yourselves. Does your home fit your new lifestyle? Patricia and Jim plan to spend at least a few years traveling much of the time. The old home might become more of a worry than a pleasure, and the stairs might pose a problem in the future should either have problems walking.

It is better to change your environment than to allow the environment to dictate what you can and cannot do. Patricia has some arthritis now. If she needed to use a walker, how would she get upstairs to her bedroom? If either of them ever needs a wheelchair, the narrow hall would be difficult to maneuver. Certainly, there would be no way to bring Patricia or Jim's elderly family members into the family home. You can sink a lot of money into a house to try to make it accommodate needs, or you can use that money for a home that is a much better fit.

If your children throw a fit about selling "our home," tell them to get over it, and they will. Now is the time to explore what housing options are available. Your goals, your needs, and your finances will be a determinant in what you choose.

Importance of Early Planning

We all need to think about what we would like to have happen if we can no longer make our own decisions. One of the best tools you can use to age successfully is a plan that you make and discuss with those in your close family circle. It is never too early to address these issues and much better to bring the family together while there is no crisis or need to make a critical decision and the elders in the family can participate.

Early planning is a gift to everyone because it avoids trying to figure out what Mom or Dad would like, and it helps to minimize the probability of family feuds with those who disagree.

We know that opening the subject of what to do when loved ones are no longer able to speak for themselves can be touchy and difficult. Do not make it about only the elders in the family. Your family may be more cooperative if you discuss what legal and health care decisions you want made for yourself and then explain that all family members need to talk about these issues and take the necessary steps to maintain their independence by letting everyone know what they want. You should discuss health care decisions, legal documents, who will handle finances, what assets are owned, and where the assets are located. With a good financial picture, then discuss the care plan, such as whether you want to stay at home or move in with a family member, or move to an assisted living facility.

If you find there is no agreement, and the meeting is disintegrating into negative territory, it may be helpful to engage a professional as a neutral facilitator. Keeping to a written agenda, moving beyond family disagreements, and suggesting resources and tools usually results in a better, more positive outcome. We suggest these meetings be held periodically to keep everyone updated.

The Caregiving Role

There is a major difference between normal aging patterns and needing care. If your loved one suffers a stroke or a fall, a serious heart ailment or a cognitive loss, care may be necessary. At that point, you may become a caregiver, and the plan will need to change. Rosalynn Carter said it best: "There are only four kinds of people in the world—those who have been caregivers, those who are currently caregivers, those who will be caregivers and those who will need caregivers."

Caregiving for another person can forge a new closeness, a higher level of understanding, and a deeper love. It can change the dynamics of your family in a positive or a negative way, but everyone will be touched by the issues that the family will face. Caregiving always involves some personal sacrifice and stress. This can manifest as exhaustion, depression, marital and family problems, or alcohol or drug abuse. You simply cannot do all the caregiving alone.

Family caregivers usually neglect their health, nutrition, and exercise routines as a result of their caregiving responsibilities. They place themselves last. It is all about the loved one in need. In spite of their sacrifice, many caregivers feel guilty. Some feel guilty because they believe they have not done enough, some because they resent taking on this life-changing challenge. Some feel guilty because they think they are not doing a good enough job, or because they lose their temper or are not being kind enough. To survive, you need to banish the guilt and acknowledge that you are doing the best you can in an ever-changing landscape.

The National Alliance for Caregiving reports that 40 to 70 percent of family caregivers have clinically significant symptoms of depression. Approximately a quarter to half of these caregivers meet the diagnostic criteria for major depression.

It is not selfish to want to continue living your life and not disappear into the caregiver role. You are not almighty. You cannot cure the problem and make it go away. You do not have all the answers. Sometimes there is no answer. You can only do the best you can.

Successful coping involves accepting what you can and cannot change. You have to let go of unrealistic expectations. If you do not, you will feel overwhelmed, guilty, and defeated. Learn to forgive yourself. This is a new situation for you, and you need to learn how to cope step by step.

The person who needs care is going through changes that may involve loss of independence and the unhappy feeling of being a burden. They may be grateful for your help, yet resentful of your hovering. They say, "leave me alone," and you say, "that's the thanks I get for sacrificing myself for you." What have you accomplished by going down that road? Both of you feel terrible. Try not to let your buttons get pushed. It is not easy but it is necessary if you do not want to be consumed by negative emotions. A sense of humor can be the best medicine.

Try not to underestimate what your loved one can do. It is often easier to perform a task for someone rather than letting him or her do it alone. Let your loved one be as independent as possible. He or she will feel more in control, less resentful, and less dependent. The time may come when you do have to step in, but let the condition decide the time, not frustration or compassion. It is hard to find that balance because you and your loved one will have good days and bad.

Aging, Dementia, and Children

Sometimes an elder relative moves into the family home, disrupting regular patterns and calling for major adjustments. It is important that all members of the family, grandkids too, understand what is going on and why this major change is happening. If you present the move as a solution and not a problem, the transition can go more smoothly. This is a great opportunity for younger members to learn firsthand about family duty, loyalty, and love. The transition requires patience, willingness to share space, and respect for privacy. Adults who grew up in a multigenerational family setting often say that the benefits outweighed the negatives, and that getting to know and learn from their elder was a great blessing. It can be hard at times, but a lifelong lesson in what families do for each other.

If your loved one has dementia, you face additional challenges. How can you explain to your children why Grandpa no longer remembers their names, or Grandma acts in a strange or frightening manner? The person they loved looks the same but is not the same. Keeping children out of what is happening will only increase their confusion and anxiety. You need to explain that dementia is a disease, and that it is the illness that has created these upsetting changes. Dementia affects the whole family unit, and each family member will have to deal with those changes, not only to their loved one, but to the family dynamic. Your children will pick up on your sadness and your stress and may model how they cope on the way you act.

Help your children understand that although they cannot cure Grandpa, a hug will go very far in making him feel loved and safe. And that they can still have a close relationship with Grandma by concentrating on not what is lost but what is still available for both of them.

Burnout

You have no doubt read and heard about burnout. It is the hopeless feeling that you simply cannot go one more day in the situation you are in, and yet, you know that you just have to. The dictionary defines burnout as an emotional condition marked by tiredness, both psychological and physical fatigue, as a result of prolonged stress. Burnout describes every caregiver at one time or another, and it is a condition that you need to preempt or create a strategy to manage.

You might be so focused on your care recipient, so determined to "fix" the situation, so aware that no matter what you do, the person continues to worsen, along with your financial situation, that you see yourself as a failure, and depression and resentment kick in.

Let's revisit Maddy and her mother, Lucy. Maddy is dealing with a mother who refuses to accept the help she needs, although she makes sure her daughter knows all the problems she is having. When Maddy pleads with her mother to let her intervene, Lucy does not thank her but tells her that she is not a child and will not be ordered around.

Lately, telephone conversations end with Maddy in tears of frustration. She loves her mother, but this is driving her mad. Maddy finally came to terms with the fact that she cannot count on her mother to change, and she does not have the power to make her mother understand. Once this "aha" moment dawned, Maddy took an aggressive step. She called her mother's minister, told him what was going on, and asked that he simply drop by and talk with her mother. If a suggestion came from someone else, maybe her mother would accept the idea. The minute Pastor Williams agreed and said he would assign a volunteer to visit Lucy regularly, Maddy felt the stress begin to dissipate. The pastor then gave Maddy some good advice.

"Maddy, you are not your mother's savior. You sound exhausted. At this point, you need more help than Lucy. Why don't you speak with your own minister and find out where and when a caregiver support group meets?"

Caregivers need to focus on themselves too. You cannot change your loved one's situation, but once you confront your own feelings, you will be able to handle the emotions you feel in a less draining way. A strong support system is essential.

If you do not reach out to family, support groups, your spiritual guide, or professional help, you will reach the point where you become a self-fulfilling prophecy, unable to function in any role and on your way to becoming ill yourself. It is sometimes hard to see yourself decompensating, but if a caring person tells you that you seem burned out, listen and get help. You must leave yourself open to making changes in your loved one's environment if you can no longer offer the care the disease demands. Do not allow yourself to be a second victim. That would be the last thing your loved one would want.

You Can Say No

It is essential to be aware of your needs and limits. You have to establish your limits and stick to them. Again, we stress the importance of the family meeting as needs progress. What you and your loved one are going through is not shameful. You will be surprised how many will share their stories once they know you are open to discussion. It is likely that some friends will drift away. The ones that stay can be a wonderful support system as needs increase. Accept the help that is offered.

CHAPTER TWO

Who Needs Eldercare?

Whether you are planning ahead or reacting to a crisis, it is important to make certain that you or your loved one's current and future medical needs will be appropriately addressed. Most diseases that affect the elderly are present in some degree throughout the general population. But some ailments affect the elderly in much greater numbers, and in this chapter, we discuss important considerations in addressing these medical concerns. We also provide some caregiving tips, including what you can do when it is no longer safe for your loved one to drive.

The Aging Process

Each person ages so individually that it is difficult to predict the physical or mental changes that may occur. Heredity, stress, diet, exercise, habits such as smoking and drinking, and even poverty play a part in the aging of a person. Everyone experiences wear and tear to organs, such as heart and lungs, as well as decreasing elasticity, especially in our skin, the largest organ of the body. There are musculoskeletal changes too. Hearing loss and changes in vision are two of most common, and more frustrating, age-related changes. It is absolutely essential to attend to these issues. A person who cannot hear well could easily misinterpret his or her environment, and an older driver with cataracts should not be behind the wheel until the medical issue is resolved.

Common Chronic Illnesses

Let's talk about the most common chronic conditions older persons may have, how they affect a person's ability to remain independent, and what steps can be taken to prevent them from interfering with a good quality of life. The most common chronic diseases afflicting the elderly are:

- adult onset diabetes
- arthritis and osteoporosis
- balance disorders
- kidney and bladder problems
- diseases of the eyes, including glaucoma, cataracts, and macular degeneration
- lung disease
- cardiovascular disease, including strokes
- depression
- dementia, including Alzheimer's disease and Parkinson's disease

Often your loved one is afraid that a diagnosis of certain conditions will mean a loss of independence. Some people will refuse to go to a physician, just hoping that everything will go away. Experts agree that one of the most practical ways you can help a loved one facing a chronic illness is by providing information about available resources to enhance their independence and quality of life. Help your loved ones understand that there are specialists and resources available to treat the illness and thus protect autonomy.

Do not skip the medical checkups. Testing and screening for diseases can catch problems that are high risk or just beginning. If disease is already present, treatment can avoid living in misery when help is available. If you are a long-distance caregiver planning a visit to your needy loved one, try not to limit your visit to the weekend only. You will miss out on visits to the doctor and other professionals you may want to meet in person.

If transportation is a problem, there are resources available to help, such as paratransit bus systems, volunteer agencies, or senior cab vouchers that will reduce the amount of a taxicab fare. We have listed these resources in appendix 2.

Adult Onset Diabetes

According the research at Johns Hopkins Bloomberg School of Public Health, the average age of elderly onset diabetes in the United States is seventy-seven years. Lifestyle factors such as an unhealthy diet, smoking, drinking, and lack of physical activity play a major role in diabetes, and conversely, living a healthful active life with good nutritional choices lessens the risk of developing diabetes. Certain medications and even bouts of depression can be risk factors for diabetes. Elderly patients need to make sure that diabetic testing is a routine part of every physician visit.

Arthritis and Osteoporosis

Arthritis is a painful inflammation of the joints that affects the musculoskeletal system. It is not a single disease but rather a term that covers more than one hundred medical conditions. Osteoarthritis is the most common form in the elderly, and this disease has no cure. It can affect the normal activities of daily living, making it extremely painful to perform tasks such as walking, bathing, dressing, and cooking. It can limit social activities, causing isolation and depression. Osteoarthritis can often be the determining factor in leaving one's home.

There are ways to assist your loved one suffering from arthritis. Physical and occupational therapists can evaluate the person's status and outline a plan of treatment to minimize the effects of the disease. Devices such as elevated toilet seats and wall bars for bathtubs will help. Get an electric can opener and a tool that can easily twist a jar top. These are examples of small adjustments that in the long run can help a person stay at home.

Balance Disorders

Falls are the leading cause of injury among elders, according to the Centers for Disease Control and Prevention. A broken hip is often the turning point in the health and quality of life of an older person. It can be the beginning of your caregiver duties and can cost the savings of a lifetime in medical care, personal home care, or a necessary alternative housing move. A serious fall can rob your loved one of most options and the ability to continue with those activities and pursuits they so enjoy.

Balance disorders are often age related. If you notice a loved one is unsteady and holds on to furniture to get around the house, make sure that problem is diagnosed and treated as soon as possible.

It is not uncommon for an elder to develop inner ear imbalance, called vestibular dysfunction. Adults with this condition are reportedly three times more likely to fall than others. If your loved one says he or she is dizzy when getting up from a prone position, find out what is causing the vertigo. High blood pressure, diabetes, or smoking could be interfering with the inner ear signaling process. Vestibular dysfunction is easily diagnosable in the doctor's office. A doctor's visit will stop the guessing game. Physical therapy can improve balance.

Sometimes a fall risk is due to frailty. Installing railings for safety will help minimize the chance of a devastating, painful, and some-times life-changing fall. Keeping rooms well lit, installing night-lights in halls and bathrooms, eliminating clutter, and painting steps and light switches with bright colors are some tips for safety in the home.

When an elderly family member refuses to acknowledge and com-pensate for serious age-related changes, it can be the beginning of a power struggle between what you see as a safety issue and he or she sees as your attempt to take away independence.

The Dreaded Fall. Lucy is described as a fiercely independent eighty-five-year-old who refuses any suggestions Maddy or her siblings make regarding the safety of her home. Lucy's home is full of scatter rugs that invite falls, but Lucy has steadfastly held on to them and would not think of picking them up or giving herself a clear passageway to walk through. She waxes her old linoleum kitchen floor until you can almost see your image in it and you don't need ice skates to slip and slide.

Her bathroom is another accident waiting to happen, with more scatter rugs and no safety bars or similar features in the bath or shower. Lucy does not understand that all her independence can be gone after a devastating fall. Maddy simply cannot dictate changes to Lucy's home, but if a health care professional discusses this issue and offers some safety recommendations, Lucy may accept the suggestions.

Maddy needs to make sure that balance issues and fall prevention are evaluated at her mother's next medical checkup. The medical exam is designed to check risk factors like poor vision, overmedication, muscle weakness, gait or balance problems, and a history of earlier falls. Perhaps the physician can suggest an exercise program for strength and balance, as well as an in-home safety assessment conducted by an occupational therapist or a geriatric care manager.

If you are trying to convince your loved one, do not make demands or become emotional. Keep the conversation light and friendly. Humor can often break the tension and may even make some sense.

Kidney and Bladder Problems

As we age, changes in the elasticity of the bladder walls can affect the efficiency of our kidneys. Certain medications, diabetes, smoking, and obesity can also put pressure on an aging organ. Urinary tract infections, bladder infections, urinary retention, and incontinence can be common occurrences in the elderly.

Incontinence is a treatable condition, but embarrassment can prevent people from seeking help. They may feel that "little accidents" are simply something one has to live with, but a physician or a nurse practitioner who specializes in treating incontinence can probably eliminate the issue or at the very least teach them to control the incontinence frequency. We will revisit this topic later.

Eye Diseases

Many older persons think that poor vision is yet another miserable but inevitable sign that they are getting older. This is not the case. It is essential for all of us, but especially the elderly, to have periodic eye exams. The earlier one detects eye disease, the better the outcome. If you keep your eye problems to yourself because you think someone may pull your driver's license and end your independence, think what blindness from an untreated condition will do to your quality of life. If you cannot see well, you can easily mix up your medication, and you will have an increased risk of falls. There are many low-vision devices, such as magnifiers, talking clocks, talking books, and the like. Specialists in low vision as well as occupational therapists can come to the home and teach ways to optimize independence. The American Foundation for the Blind is a national nonprofit that expands possibilities for people with vision loss.

Lung Disease

Chronic obstructive pulmonary disease (COPD) is a term used to describe a group of progressive respiratory disorders that are often the product of elderly lungs with decreased elasticity. Smoking is a major factor in the development of COPD. Pneumonia, an infection of the lungs, is a major cause of mortality among people aged sixty-five and older. It is harder for elders to fight off infections because of weaker immune systems. Other health conditions, such as any neurodegenerative disease, or frailty can make pneumonia dangerous. It is recommended that elders get an annual flu shot and the one-time pneumococcal vaccine. If you are a caregiver, be sure to have the shots yourself to ensure that you do not get ill or pass anything on to your loved one.

If your loved one needs oxygen, get portable tanks as well as the standard size. A small tank ensures that life need not be tethered to a big tank. If your loved one is frightened about not being able to breathe, ask for an antianxiety medication to control the level of fear. Exercise, relaxation techniques, and social activities are wonderful ways to help a person cope with breathing issues. Medical treatment from a specialist in pulmonary diseases is also important.

Cardiovascular Disease, Including Stroke

Elders that suffer from high blood pressure, heart disease, diabetes, and the effects of smoking, too much alcohol, or obesity are at high risk for stroke. A stroke happens when a blood clot blocks an artery or a blood vessel breaks. As a result, brain cells begin to die, and the abilities controlled by that part of the brain are lost. Depending on which part of the brain is attacked, speech, memory, or movement will be damaged. Getting your loved one medical attention immediately after or during a stroke is of the utmost importance. You must learn the symptoms and then act.

The sad truth is that stoke victims wait sometimes days before seeking medical care, and by then the damage may be irreparable. Post-stroke treatment may include physical and occupational therapy, often as an inpatient. Your loved one may need to call on you or a paid caregiver as he or she recuperates or learns to live with permanent post-stroke disabilities. As a caregiver, you need to educate yourself and your loved one about the disability and how best to avoid a reoccurrence. You need to learn about resources that can assist you financially, practically, and emotionally.

Depression

Depression in the elderly is a widespread problem, but it is not a normal part of aging. It is often not recognized or treated. Some signs of depression include being sad more often than not, losing interest in everything, sleeping too much or not at all, eating too much or having no desire for food. Any number of things can trigger a depressive mode. Elders often face the loss of their home and sometimes a move far away or to a facility; they often suffer from illness or pain. They may mourn the loss of a beloved spouse, child, or even a dear pet, all leading to feelings of giving up. Some medications can trigger depression, and neuro-degenerative dementia can have a depression modality.

The good news is that depression often responds to treatment. If you can get your loved one to a geriatric health care professional for treatment, many medications and therapies can be extremely helpful. Social activities, along with love and support from family and a professionally led support group, will accelerate the successful treatment of this disease.

If your loved one says he or she is contemplating suicide, take it seriously. Take control of the medications and get rid of weapons, be they guns, sharp instruments, or household poisons. Nevada ranks among the highest in the country for elder suicide. Older adults who live alone, who have access to guns, and who have not been treated for diagnosable clinical depression are at highest risk. If you have to walk your loved one into an emergency room to get the help, do it. If there is no cooperation, call 911 and explain the situation. Do not allow your loved one to become another suicide statistic.

Dementia

With aging as a high risk factor, many people face dementia. The statistics are chilling. The Social Security Administration estimates that 25 percent of those who are now sixty-five years old will live past age ninety, and an estimated one in eight persons past age sixty-five has Alzheimer's disease. Along with increased life span comes a dramatic increase in the prevalence of Alzheimer's disease. It is the sixth leading cause of death in the United States.

Another staggering statistic is that unpaid caregivers—in other words, family caregivers—provide about 17.4 billion hours of care to persons with Alzheimer's disease and other dementias. In 2012, services to beneficiaries with Alzheimer's disease and other dementias cost Medicare and Medicaid an estimated 140 billion dollars.

The word dementia comes from the Latin *de,* meaning "apart," and *mens,* meaning "mind." The great disconnect has been described as a "loss of self." Dementia is a degenerative, progressive neurological disorder (i.e., a neurodegenerative disorder) that involves significant loss of intellectual ability, such as memory, that is severe enough to interfere with normal functioning. Alzheimer's disease is the most common form of dementia but there are other progressive, incurable types of dementias.

Vascular cognitive impairment, dementia with Lewy body, Parkinson disease, frontal temporal dementia (known as Pick's disease), HIV dementia, and Creutzfeldt-Jakob disease are some that fall into this category. It is possible that someone may have a "mixed" dementia, having developed more than one type of the disorder.

Symptoms that appear to be dementia could be due to a treatable condition, such as overmedication. Elders take more medication than any other part of the population. Too many medications, both prescription and over the counter; poor nutrition; dehydration; and even a urinary tract infection can look like dementia.

If the person's cognitive impairment is from a brain tumor, subdural hematoma, normal pressure hydrocephalus, vitamin B12 deficiency, or low levels of thyroid, known as hypothyroidism, the dementia can be treated. Even depression can mask as dementia, sending the person and the family down the wrong path.

All medical possibilities must be checked to ensure the correct diagnosis. We suggest starting with the primary physician, then obtaining a referral to a geriatrician, a neurologist specializing in dementia, or a geriatric psychiatrist. Nevada is fortunate to have the Cleveland Clinic Lou Ruvo Center for Brain Health in Las Vegas and in Elko. This center is fast becoming renowned for the treatment of neurodegenerative diseases. The Cleveland Clinic describes their services as patient focused and multidisciplined for the diagnosis and treatment of cognitive disorders. It is a center for research, education, and support services for family members.

Alzheimer's Disease

Contrary to the myth that Alzheimer's disease is inevitable as one ages, it is not a normal part of aging, although it is the most common form of dementia, especially in the elderly. At this time, the disease is progressive, meaning the symptoms and cognitive impairment will get worse with time. Early symptoms of Alzheimer's include difficulty remembering names and recent events, apathy, mood swings, and depression. As the disease progresses, patients often exhibit disorientation and severe impairments in walking, speaking, and swallowing.

The victims of this disease will lose more memory, experience increased confusion, often forget their vocabulary, lose the ability to make decisions, forget their loved ones, and in essence lose themselves. Currently, there is no treatment other than medications that may slow the progress of the disease.

This devastating disease is a family affair. Every member of the family is affected, and the lives of those close to the care receiver will change forever. Caregivers can only watch as the disease progresses, erasing memories and abilities to function normally. The process is frustrating, heartbreaking, and deeply sad. This disease can bring a family close or tear it apart.

Tips for Handling Dementia and Alzheimer's Disease. If your loved one has a neurodegenerative disease, then being reasonable and logical will not work. You can never win an argument with a person who has dementia. Judgment skills and memory no longer play a part in his or her life. Your loved one lives in a different reality, and the ability to understand and remember is mostly gone. If you ask your loved one not to ever do something again, or to remember to do something, it will soon be forgotten.

For people who have mild cognitive impairment or early stage dementia, leaving notes as reminders can sometimes help, but as the dementia progresses, this will not work and may even cause more confusion.

Taking action to make the environment safer, rather than talking and discussing, is usually a more successful approach. For example, getting a tea kettle with an automatic off switch is better than warning someone of the dangers of leaving the stove on. Removing the locks on all bathroom doors will prevent your loved one getting locked in and pounding to get out. It will also allow you access if the person does not respond to your knocks, or if you see water seeping under the door. You may want to install an automatic shutoff on the faucets and a governor on the hot water faucet to avoid a mishap.

Keep things simple. The less change, the better. Do not purchase a new microwave that is "easier" to use. It won't be. Your loved one will not be able to learn anything new. It is better to keep the old appliance and label what is confusing.

The Alzheimer's Association offers the Safe Return bracelet. Safe Return is a nationwide identification, support, and registration program working at the community level. The program provides assistance whether a person becomes lost locally or far from home. Assistance is available twenty-four hours, every day, whenever a person is lost or found. The person wears an engraved identification bracelet with an 800 telephone number on the bracelet. Safe Return can access the registrant information and notify listed contacts. You can install alarms on the doors to avoid a crisis with wandering. You can also install an emergency response system in the home for you to have in case something happens to you and your loved one can no longer call for help. As best you can, plan ahead.

Case Study: The Petersons

Jim and Patricia Peterson have become very worried about Jim's dad, George, given the reports of his problems with driving and his repetitive telephone conversations. They decide to visit George and get a first-hand look at what is happening. On top of the worry over her father-in-law, Patricia is getting concerned about her husband. Jim seems so distracted lately.

They have a circle of friends they see often, and lately she has had to whisper to Jim, "You told that story before." He sometimes admits he is having a tough time remembering and that his job is getting harder and harder for him to do. She chalks it up to boredom and maybe anxiety about his retirement future. She is really glad he has only a few months more of work.

When Jim and Patricia arrive at George's home in Reno, they are shocked. The place is filthy, the sink full of dirty dishes, and the bathroom overflowed. George had forgotten about their visit and seems confused about almost everything. He looks like he has lost a great deal of weight and is as unkempt as the house. Patricia notices a stack of overdue bills, and when she asks George about them, he hits the roof and wants to know why she is stealing his money. Patricia also observes several prescription bottles, all expired and most full of medication. Patricia shows Jim all the dents and scrapes on George's car and the five traffic tickets for moving violations that George was ignoring.

Try as she might, Patricia cannot get a straight answer from George, and although her husband is upset, he seems to distance himself from the disaster and simply sits with his dad in front of the television to watch baseball. The neighbor comes to the door and tells Jim and Patricia that she tried and tried to help, but when George became angry and aggressive, she backed off. That is the reason she called Jim and Patricia and begged them to come quickly, because something was really wrong.

The Petersons had not gotten their legal papers in order. They were going to handle all that after Jim's retirement. Now all those plans have gone away, and at age fifty-three, Patricia's life has taken an unexpected turn. It dawns on her that she is on her own and that she very likely does not have one needy person but two. If Patricia does not ask for help and support, she could burn out. It is time to call the family for whatever support they can offer.

Taking Away the Keys

There may come a time when it is no longer safe for you or your loved one to drive. If Mom is having fender benders, if Dad goes through stop signs, if changing lanes safely is becoming a problem, acknowledge those warning signs. Medications, failing eye sight, dementia, arthritis, and slowed ability to make quick decisions all play a role in risky behavior behind the wheel.

Many older drivers try to compensate by avoiding highways or nighttime driving, yet drivers over age seventy are more likely than younger drivers to be involved in accidents. Older drivers are more likely to have fatal crashes, and a vast percentage occur during daytime hours. Not every older driver is dangerous. Performance trumps statistics.

It does not matter whether your loved one lives in the city or in the rural part of the state, even the thought of losing the use of a car is a blow to independence and autonomy. It affects the ability to make appointments and spontaneous plans, or to just go to the store for the weekly groceries. Simple tasks become difficult for you and for your loved one. You have to arrange your life around the transportation needs of your loved one. If you live at a distance, you may have to hire someone to be on call to drive.

Can you imagine how hard it is to rely on others for rides to the supermarket, to necessary appointments, or to visit friends and family? Depression and isolation are common side effects of not being able to drive. The care provider may begin to resent the extra burden even though the need is clear.

When you are making your care plans, you have to address this subject. You need to start this conversation before there is an issue. Talking about some of the risks for older drivers and the red flags they can look for themselves is a great help. Suggest taking a driver safety course. AARP has an in-person and an online course that teaches how to be a better, safer driver, available for those over age fifty. Do it together and the threatening aspect of the subject will disappear. For some, the possibility of a discount on car insurance will tip the scale.

Dementia and Driving

In the early stages of Alzheimer's disease, it is possible for someone to continue driving short distances to familiar places. Use the "children" test. Ask yourself if you would let your children or grandchildren ride with your loved one behind the wheel. If the answer is "no," you must step in.

Remember this is a progressive disease, and your loved one cannot be the judge of when to give up the keys. This may be one of the big battles that you simply have to win for the safety of your relative and everyone else. Start transitioning the driver away from the driver role so that when it is absolutely necessary, the loss of that role may not be so big a jolt. You may need to call on a neutral professional to convince your loved one that he or she can no longer drive. Occupational therapists with specialized training can perform a comprehensive driving assessment.

You may have to hide the keys or, if you have two cars, remove one. Then you will be the driver of the only car, and you alone will possess the keys. Do not leave them in your pocket or hanging up on a hook. You may wake up one day to find your loved one and car long gone.

If driving becomes an issue that you cannot solve on your own, tell your loved one's doctor. The physician can send a confidential physician's report to the Department of Motor Vehicles recommending that the driver's license be revoked.

Community Resources

Educate yourself about whatever caregiving issue you are dealing with and find out what services and resources are available. You need to have time away from caregiving. Do not let your activities and interests slide away. You have a right, even a responsibility, to let someone step in to help. Find out about adult daycare or in-home caregivers, from an agency, a private caregiver referred to you from a reliable source, or volunteers through nonprofit agencies like Helping Hands or Catholic Charities.

Respite Care

A little respite can relieve some of your stress, but another aspect of respite care is important—giving your loved one a break from you too. Your loved one needs to know that even if you are away, he or she will be safe. If you become the shadow of your loved one, it will be that much more traumatic if you need to find alternative placement.

Having some time away, in a group setting, enables your loved one to socialize and make friends. It is empowering for both of you. You may have to insist at first, but taking some time apart soon becomes fun and rewarding.

Support Groups

Whether you are a primary or a long-distance caregiver for an aging relative, or if someone you love has dementia, one of the best things you can do for yourself and for your loved one is to attend a support group. A support group lessens the feeling of isolation and despair that often comes with the responsibility of taking on the care of another person.

The group understands and is nonjudgmental, sharing valuable tips. A support group can give you back that sense of control you need to complete the journey. What a relief to be in a setting where people "get it." You will find friends to share the burden, and you will learn about resources that will help ease the load.

Some support groups offer respite care and supervised socialization for loved ones during the meeting. If you cannot attend a group in person, online groups provide a place for caregivers to share feelings and information.

If, for some reason, you simply cannot attend a group or feel uncomfortable in a group setting, do not just close the door on sharing your feelings. Keep a journal, talk to a good friend, seek counsel through your church, synagogue, mosque, or a professional therapist, but let it out.

Just as it is vital for you to meet and share with others who have similar difficulties, your loved one can benefit from a confidential setting to express fears and other feelings. Receiving support from others is a powerful tool for everyone.

CHAPTER THREE

There's No Place Like Home

The goal of eldercare is to allow you or your loved ones to live safely, comfortably, and stress free in familiar surroundings for as long as possible.

Lucy has lived in Elko, Nevada, all her life. She was baptized in the church she still attends. Her parents and siblings are buried in the church cemetery, and Lucy will tell anyone who listens that she intends to leave her house feet first and not a day before. Lucy has arthritis, kidney problems, and high blood pressure. She suffers in silence from incontinence, the one condition she has not shared with anyone. For all those like Lucy and those who care for them, following are some tips for helping your loved one stay at home as long as possible.

Keeping the Home Safe
Halls and Doorways

- Make sure all rugs have nonskid backing and remove those that do not.
- Keep pathways clear.
- Get everything off the floor to avoid tripping.
- Make sure all cords are out of the way.
- Place furniture where it does not present a fall risk.
- If possible, widen doorways so a walker or wheelchair will fit. See if removing a door completely might help.

Bathroom Safety Tips

- Install grab bars in the shower and tub to avoid slips. If possible, install a grab bar next to the toilet or install a raised toilet seat.
- Use a nonskid surface or rubber mat in the shower or bathtub.
- Use a shower chair to reduce slips and install a handheld shower head if needed.
- Install nightlights to guide the way to the bathroom as well as in the bathroom.

Kitchen Safety Tips

- Check the stove and change the handles if turning them is a problem.
- Make sure the stove area is free of clutter.
- Make sure the kitchen mat is nonskid.
- If pots are too heavy, switch to lighter ones.
- Rearrange shelves to avoid using ones that cannot be reached safely.
- Use special arthritis-friendly implements, like jar and bottle openers or reachers.
- If there is a stepstool, make sure it is steady. Do not use a step-stool with more than two steps.
- If you or your loved one enjoys cooking, but standing is making cooking difficult, try a steady, high chair for taking frequent breaks. If you or your loved one does not enjoy cooking, think of using prepared meals.
- If shopping is an issue, many of the big chain supermarkets provide food delivery service. Consider hiring home health caregivers to help with shopping and preparing meals.
- If housebound through a temporary illness or a permanent condition, contact the local "Meals on Wheels" program. Low-cost meals are home delivered.
- Make sure the smoke alarm is working in the kitchen area and throughout the home.

Bedroom Safety Tips

- Make sure the bedroom light can be turned on before entering the room.
- A remote control device can make it easy to turn off an overhead light or fan without getting out of bed.
- Make sure a lamp is within easy reach of the bedside.
- Install nightlights to guide the way to the bathroom.
- Install an automatic lift for the bed if necessary.

Stair Tips

- Make sure the banisters are sturdy.
- Install a light switch at the top and at the bottom of the stairs.
- Check the carpeting or install rubber treads on each step.
- Install an automatic lift for stairs if necessary.

The Cost of "Aging in Place"

Many of the products we suggest are inexpensive and can easily be obtained at your local hardware or home improvement store. Another good way to get such items as jar openers and pill box dispensers is to attend a health fair. You will come home with many items that can be helpful around the house.

Some of the more expensive devices, such as wheelchairs, walkers, and the like are covered by insurance with an accompanying prescription from a primary physician. If your loved one has had a hospital visit, the discharge planner can arrange for hospital beds, commodes, and other necessary medical equipment. The discharge planner can also arrange for home visits for physical therapy, occupational therapy, and home health for a few months. Check with your or your loved one's insurance carrier to see what they do and do not cover.

Emergency Response System

In an emergency, time is of the essence. If someone is having chest pain, or has fallen and cannot get up, an emergency response system can save a life.

This device will give twenty-four-hour emergency help just by pushing a button worn on the person. Trained operators answer any call and are ready to send emergency help, by requesting an ambulance, calling the fire department, or simply contacting a neighbor or family member who can then check. The cost of this system varies from company to company, but the monthly rental is not expensive, and some supplemental insurance benefits cover emergency response costs. Check with your or your loved one's insurance carrier.

Medical History Bracelet

A medical history bracelet has an individual's medical history loaded into a memory device located in the band. The bracelet plugs directly to a USB so that this medical history and other information will be immediately accessible. You can take it wherever you go, and most are waterproof. It is easy for a caregiver to add and delete information to keep the device up to date.

More Resources

Other ways to accommodate the needs of loved ones include big button cell phones, doorbell-telephone flashing-light signaler for the hard of hearing, automatic pill reminders, and monitoring systems. If this seems overwhelming to you, enlist the services of an eldercare specialist or geriatric care manager to assess the home and make specific recommendations with reliable resource names.

Tips for Handling Incontinence

When clients tell us their eldercare challenges, they often lower their voice in embarrassment when mentioning incontinence. Sometimes they will even seek placement outside the home just because of incontinence. Some conditions are just plain embarrassing and therefore never addressed. So many older persons are struggling with this issue, yet they often do not seek treatment. Many cases are treatable.

Urinary incontinence is any involuntary loss of urine. This issue is so sensitive that it can play havoc with an elder's quality of life and cause him or her to withdraw from social activities for fear of offending. Studies show women wait three years before seeking treatment, and men wait about six months. This is generally because most women have worn maxi-pads, so they are more comfortable purchasing incontinence pads and even adult diapers than they are talking to a medical doctor about "leaking."

There are two types of incontinence: acute, which appears during an illness or specific medical problem, and persistent, or chronic, which occurs because of issues with function of the lower urinary tract. For example, dehydration, infection, or certain medications or combinations of medications can cause acute incontinence. Once the underlying condition is resolved, the incontinence usually disappears. Neurological impairment, such as dementia, can eliminate the perception of the need to urinate.

Chronic incontinence is generally categorized as stress, urge, or mixed. Stress incontinence is when leakage occurs during coughing, sneezing, or physical activity. Urge incontinence is sometimes called the "key in the lock" syndrome. You need to go badly, you are almost home, you put that key in the lock, and you cannot hold it anymore.

Behavioral therapy, bladder training, and change in fluid intake and diet are remarkably helpful. Pelvic floor muscle exercises, generally known as Kegels, help strengthen the muscles that aging and other issues have made weak. Medications can also help. Treatment of incontinence is highly successful. Get professional help. The more you know and share with your loved one, the more control he or she will have, which in turn improves quality of life.

CHAPTER FOUR

Planning for the Cost of Long-Term Care

Maybe you are trying to figure out the best living situation for yourself, or maybe you are helping someone else plan for or manage long-term care. Most people who need assistance with daily living receive it unpaid from family and friends. But many people pay for the care they receive, either at home, in an assisted living facility, or in a nursing home. The next several chapters explain what you can do to protect and preserve assets.

This chapter focuses on the different arrangements for care, and how to maximize your financial situation to privately cover the cost. Various programs and insurance may also help pay for the care.

Nursing homes are expensive, and without careful planning, a long-term stay in one can wipe out the life savings of most families. The average cost of a nursing home in Nevada is $7,200 a month. If your loved one needs care for three years, the cost is over $250,000. In chapter 5 we explain how you may be able to qualify for Medicaid coverage of your nursing home bills, without losing everything, according to the law in Nevada. That chapter covers the income rules and asset rules, and explains what you can do under Nevada law to protect your assets.

Are you aware of the benefit for veterans who qualify that will give a monthly allowance to elderly veterans and their spouses even without a service-connected disability? In chapter 6, we explain how you may be able to obtain veterans' benefits to help pay for the cost of care.

Without proper legal advice, many people spend down their assets to the level of Medicaid eligibility. In most cases, people spend more than is required, jeopardizing the financial security of a spouse and leaving them without the ability to pay for items and extras not covered by the Medicaid program. Many clients who come to our office in crisis mode are surprised to learn that they will have no ability to pay for simple things like clothes, hearing aids, or special foods.

Also, many clients with children express the strong desire to be able to pass on a part of their life savings to their children, and most wish to pass on the family home. Those clients without children usually want to give some of their assets to other family members, rather than using it all on a nursing home.

Medicaid is a joint state and federal program. The federal government sets basic requirements, but each state may implement them differently, so the programs vary greatly from state to state. This book focuses specifically on Nevada law so that you know what works in Nevada at the time of this book's printing. Medicaid and veterans' benefits are both complex areas, and the rules are constantly changing. Always consult a qualified attorney to go over your situation. Your facts and circumstances can differ from others, and your values and goals may necessitate a different planning strategy.

Once you become aware of the planning possibilities available to you, you can avoid the kinds of transfers or mistakes that can get you in trouble and that can be avoided with proper knowledge. Every technique and option in this book is legal. Simply "hiding" money is not an option. It is fraud, with severe legal consequences. Long-term care planning is permitted under law. If the government does not like these options, they will change the law, which they regularly do. We have found that some people feel comfortable with every available legal planning technique; others do not. You should be aware of the laws and planning strategies available under federal law and Nevada law so that you can decide which techniques are right for you.

Types of Care

The number of elderly in the United States is growing at a rapid rate. According to the federal Administration on Aging, by the year 2030 more than 85 million people will be over age sixty, with 9 million over age eighty-five. Modern medicine and scientific breakthroughs are prolonging our lives. Many in our aging population are active people who contribute to the culture, economy, and stability of society. But, with increased lifespans, more elderly are requiring assistance for a longer period.

More care options are available now than at any time in the past. The government and private industry have responded to the increased demand for services with more home-oriented services, assisted living alternatives, community-based services, and caregiver services. More alternatives mean more choices to make. For example:

- Aging in place. The loved one remains in his or her lifelong place of residence and receives assistance from outside service providers or from family members.
- Living with family. The loved one moves in with a family member who can more readily and conveniently provide the assistance the loved one requires.
- Assisted living facilities or group homes. These residential facilities combine some of the advantages of independent life with ready access to assistance with the activities of daily living.
- Long-term care nursing facilities or skilled nursing facilities. Nursing homes provide round-the-clock care for individuals who cannot care for themselves and whose level of necessary care is beyond the abilities of a family member or assisted living facility.

Many people strongly resist the idea of entering a nursing home. Many adult children promise they will do all they can to avoid that option, but the time may come when a nursing home is the only viable choice. Such a facility is needed for elders who require twenty-four-hour nursing care far above what another type of facility can offer. Most nursing facilities accept Medicaid. Once your loved one has been approved for Medicaid, virtually all your medical bills will be paid by the program. This includes prescription drugs, hospital stays, and the nursing home bill, less your small portion. Most people keep their Medicare coverage, which may overlap.

If your loved one is living at home or in an assisted living facility, Medicaid refers to this as living "in the community." Nevada has a home and community–based waiver program, which has different rules for qualification. These services often have a waiting list, but if your loved one becomes eligible and is selected, the program may pay for care in contracted group homes and assisted living facilities, or pay for limited in-home care.

Paying for Care

There are five ways to pay the cost of long-term care.

1. Pay with your own funds. This is the method many people are required to use at first. Quite simply, it means paying for the cost of a nursing home out of your own pocket. Unfortunately, with nursing home bills averaging $7,200 per month in our area, few people can afford a long-term stay in a nursing home.

2. Long-term care insurance. If you are fortunate enough to have this type of coverage, it may go a long way toward paying the cost of the nursing home. Unfortunately, long-term care insurance is expensive, and most people facing a nursing home stay do not have this coverage.

3. Medicare. Medicare is the national health insurance program primarily for people age sixty-five years or older, certain younger disabled people, and people with kidney failure. Medicare provides only short-term assistance with nursing home costs, and only if strict qualification rules are met.

4. Medicaid. Medicaid is a federal- and state-funded, state-administered medical benefit program that can pay for the cost of nursing home care if certain asset and income requirements are met.

5. Veterans' benefits. Veterans' benefits for qualified veterans and surviving spouses help pay for the cost of long-term care if specific rules are met. Veterans' benefits are governed solely by federal law.

Long-Term Care Insurance

Long-term care insurance provides some protection against the cost of long-term care. In determining whether to purchase long-term care insurance, you have to consider its cost over many years, the likelihood that you will need enough paid care to make it worthwhile, and the specific policies available to you.

If you are shopping for a long-term care insurance policy, do not choose solely based on premium. Select a reputable company by first checking the company's reliability rating. You should not rely on the brochure or summary, but instead take the time to examine the entire policy. Take it home and study it carefully.

You must be eligible to attain a policy, which means you will have to provide information about your current health and health history. Depending on your medical history and condition, plus your age, the insurance company may not offer you a policy. Or they might charge you a considerably higher premium because of your age or health history.

You should also analyze the cost of premiums, and consider that premiums are likely to rise throughout the life of the policy. Financial planners generally recommend that you not purchase long-term care insurance if the premiums are more than 5 percent of your income.

The cost of care increases over time, so consider purchasing inflation protection, which will raise your benefit amount over the years. Inflation protection increases the cost of premiums, but it is essential. Other terms and conditions in your policy can mean higher or lower premiums.

What About Medicare?

There is a great deal of confusion about Medicare and Medicaid. Medicare is a federal health insurance program primarily for people over age sixty-five as well as disabled persons to pay for hospital and other medical services. Some limited long-term care benefits may be available under Medicare. In general, if a person is enrolled in the traditional Medicare plan and has a hospital stay of at least three days before being admitted into a skilled nursing facility for rehabilitation or skilled nursing care, Medicare may pay for a while. If the person is a Medicare Managed Care Plan beneficiary, a three-day hospital stay may not be required to qualify.

If your loved one is sent to the hospital in an emergency situation, make sure an overnight stay is classified as an admission and not "under observation." If a hospital stay is classified as an observation, the patient can be ineligible for various Medicare benefits. More than 1.5 million Medicare hospital stays in 2012 were classified as observation visits. As a result, Medicare implemented a rule that doctors should admit as inpatients those they expect to stay in the hospital for two or more nights. Sometimes families learn that Medicare will not cover the cost of rehabilitation in a skilled nursing stay because their loved one was not considered an inpatient for at least three days. This can add up to thousands of dollars, so be sure to check the status of the hospital stay and, if necessary, get the admitting doctor to change to an inpatient status before discharge.

If certain qualifications are met, Medicare may pay the full cost of the nursing home stay for the first twenty days, then continue to pay the nursing home stay for the next eighty days but with a deductible of more than one hundred dollars per day. Some Medicare supplemental insurance policies will pay the cost of the deductible.

In the best-case scenario, Medicare may pay up to one hundred days for each "spell of illness." To qualify for one hundred days of coverage, however, the nursing home resident must be receiving daily "skilled care." Once the nursing home resident requires only custodial care, Medicare will not pay. (Note: Once the Medicare and Managed Care beneficiary has not received a Medicare-covered level of care for sixty consecutive days, the beneficiary may again be eligible for the one hundred days of skilled nursing coverage for the next spell of illness.)

The difference between skilled care and custodial care is crucial. Care is considered custodial if a lay person can perform it without special professional training, such as helping someone dress, eat, or bathe.

Medicare covers daily skilled care and rehabilitative services provided in a Medicare-certified skilled nursing facility. A patient is not required to be capable of recovery or even improvement for the services to be covered. Physical therapy to prevent deterioration is enough to justify skilled care.

When a skilled nursing facility believes a service is not covered by Medicare, it must inform you in writing. You have the right to demand that the facility bill Medicare, and you do not have to pay for the service until Medicare denies payment. When Medicare denies payment, you have the right to appeal that decision, but you must pay for the services pending the appeal.

Medicare offers prescription drug coverage to everyone it covers. If you decide not to join a Medicare prescription drug plan when you are first eligible, and you do not have other creditable prescription drug coverage, you will likely pay a late enrollment penalty if you do end up needing coverage. To obtain Medicare drug coverage, you must join a plan run by an insurance company or other private company approved by Medicare. Each plan can vary in cost and drugs covered.

Assess Medical Needs and Personal Needs

Because a specific physical or mental condition often leads to the need for long-term care, one of the first things you should do is get professional advice about the need for immediate care and about likely changes in the condition over time. Talk with your primary care physician, who may refer you to a specialist. The health care professional can discuss the level of care that would be required to deliver those medical services, whether to anticipate a short or long recovery period, and whether a condition is likely to stabilize or become worse over time.

You will need to address what personal, nonmedical care is needed and what aspects of daily life a person can still manage without outside assistance. Some people are fiercely independent and private. Others prefer the security and ease of care provided by others. The solution for each will often be different.

What Can You Afford?

Nevada has a wide variety of group homes and residential facilities. Home care is also an option, but if more than part-time care is needed, the expense generally exceeds that of care in a group home or residential facility. The cost varies depending on the facility and often increases over time. In general, independent living facilities average $1,500 per month, assisted living facilities average $2,500 per month, and memory care facilities average $4,000 per month. Whatever the initial rate is when you select the facility, that rate will often increase as your loved one requires more care. Nursing homes average $7,200 per month. Most licensed and bonded home health care workers cost around twenty dollars per hour, which totals more than $14,000 per month for twenty-four-hour daily care.

Determine Income and Assets

The first step in determining what money is available for someone's long-term care is to add up that person's income and available assets, less any liabilities. When social security was established in the 1930s, it was usually described as one leg of a three-legged stool to support retirees. The first leg was supposed to be private savings, and the second was private pension. Social security was intended to ensure that even poor retirees would have a minimum of support. In practice, the three-legged stool has been completely upset. Many seniors depend almost entirely on social security. Private pensions have become a relative rarity, and with changes in the economy, the few remaining are less stable. In addition to social security and pension benefits, some seniors may have income from rental property, investments, or other sources.

The most common assets are cash, savings, money-market accounts, checking accounts, certificates of deposit, bonds, brokerage accounts, stocks, real property, vehicles, life insurance, and personal property.

Some families will offer financial support to other family members. A survey found that 62 percent of adult children caregivers say the cost of caring for a parent has affected their ability to plan for their own financial future. Long-term care costs are not the only expenses caregivers bear. In addition to providing hands-on care, family members often reach into their own pockets to pay for many daily expenses, including groceries, household goods, prescription drugs, medical copayments, and transportation.

Financing Home Care Through Reverse Mortgages

Many seniors have no long-term care insurance coverage and do not have enough income and liquid assets to pay for their care at home. Many own their home outright, or have considerable equity in their home. Seniors may be able to convert their home equity into cash while continuing to live at home as long as they are able to do so. A reverse mortgage is a loan against the value of the home paid as a lump sum, monthly amount, line of credit, or some combination. This loan does not have to be repaid until the borrower sells or otherwise permanently leaves the home.

Because the money received is a loan, it is not taxable as income, nor does it count against social security benefits if the recipient has not reached full retirement age. When the borrower sells the home, he or she must pay back the loan out of the proceeds. If the borrower dies or permanently leaves the home, such as to move into an assisted living facility, the lender must be repaid within a certain time, usually one year to eighteen months. This often means the borrower or the estate will have to sell the house to repay the reverse mortgage. If the property is sold for more than the amount of the mortgage, then the owner or the owner's survivors keep the difference. If the property is sold for less than the amount of the mortgage, neither the owner nor the survivors have to take the loss.

Reverse mortgages have drawbacks. They often have high initial fees, closing costs, origination costs, and service charges. If the recipient dies or moves out of the home before drawing much on the mortgage, he or she winds up paying a very high cost for what turned out to be a short-term loan. Continuing fees and interest payments each year lessen the money actually received. Further, interest compounds under a reverse mortgage, so that interest is paid on interest as the loan period goes on. This means that over years, a modest initial reverse mortgage can cost considerably more than other forms of borrowing.

All government-insured loans require potential borrowers to receive counseling from a financial adviser not connected to the lending institution. The adviser can explain the loan details and discuss the advantages and disadvantages. If you are considering a non-government-insured loan, you should seek an independent adviser not connected with the lending institution.

AARP recommends asking yourself five questions before you take the next step on a reverse mortgage.

1. *Have I investigated less costly options?* Look very carefully at alternatives, including a home equity loan, downsizing, selling, and moving. You may prefer to live in a different place at a lower cost. If you are a wartime veteran or a widow of a wartime veteran, investigate aid and attendance benefits to help pay for home care.

2. *How long do I expect to stay in my home?* The up-front costs are so high that if you plan to move in a few years, a reverse mortgage is probably not the best solution. Circumstances can unexpectedly upend plans. If you are older and need funds to pay for in-home health care or to make ends meet to remain at home, it could make sense.

3. *Do I need the loan now?* The danger with taking a reverse mortgage too soon is that your nest egg would not be there down the road, when you might really need it.

4. *Should I invest the money from a reverse mortgage?* According to AARP, the answer is no. The loan would cost you more than you could safely earn. Be wary of anyone who tries to sell you something and suggests using a reverse mortgage to pay for it.

5. *Have I discussed this plan with family?* Consider talking with your family about your concerns. According to AARP, in many

cases, the children suggest the reverse mortgage in the first place, but the family should understand the effect on the estate.

Cashing in Life Insurance

Life insurance policies offer another source of funds for seniors who are terminally ill. By cashing in a life insurance policy, a senior can receive a substantial amount of money relatively quickly, without having to worry about how the money will be paid back. There are many drawbacks. The amount received will be considerably less than the policy's face value, which is the amount that would have been paid to the beneficiary at the death of the insured.

The amount received may make you ineligible for Medicaid benefits to pay for nursing home care. Medicaid does not consider the face value of a life insurance policy as an asset, nor does it require you to cash in a term policy. But if you do cash it in, it is an available asset. If you are using the funds to pay for care at home or another care setting that Medicaid would not cover, then this will not be a drawback.

Some life insurance policies may be cashed in directly with the insurance company itself, a procedure known as collecting accelerated or living benefits. If the policy provides for accelerated benefits, it usually requires a physician to declare the policyholder terminally ill. Read the terms of your policy carefully.

If you do not qualify for accelerated benefits, you can make a life settlement of your policy. Life settlement companies pay a lump sum to a life insurance policyholder under certain circumstances. The younger and healthier the person selling the life insurance, the lower the settlement. The company that buys the policy pays the premiums, and then the proceeds are paid to the company at the death of the policy holder. Check to make sure the company is licensed to conduct business in your state. It is also a good idea to consult with an independent accountant, lawyer, or financial adviser.

Avoiding Common Financial Mistakes

If you have time to plan for long-term care, one important way is to engage in careful financial planning. This means avoiding common mistakes that can unnecessarily reduce the amount of funds available for care.

- Not using a qualified professional. Unless you have a family member who is an accountant or a certified financial planner, you should seek outside professional help for managing your money. There is nothing wrong with letting your loved ones know that their advice is appreciated, but make sure you double-check their suggestions with a trusted and trained financial expert.
- Having an inadequate long- and short-term plan. Few Americans have developed a financial plan to see them through retirement. Lacking a healthy perspective of inflation and how it may affect your future purchasing power can leave you with too little money for future care. You need to make sure that your investments, social security income, and so forth more than keep pace with inflation. Without a plan for the future, you may also find yourself in a situation where you spend too much of your liquid assets too soon.
- Becoming vulnerable to scams and exploitation. Statistics show that one in five Americans older than sixty-five have been preyed on by scammers, who are constantly coming up with new ways to cheat the people they feel are most vulnerable. The elderly always top the list of a swindler's potential victims. You need to be vigilant against scammers. Exploitation can severely deplete assets available for long-term care. A desperate or needy family member is often the one to take advantage of the senior, leaving the senior with nothing for his or her own care.

Having the foresight to make arrangements for long-term care can save the rest of the family emotional and financial distress. For those who lack the resources, or who did not plan ahead, the next chapters discuss some options to access benefits.

Tax Issues Related to Long-Term Care

Many people want to know whether the cost of care paid privately, such as payment to an assisted living facility or to family and friends, can be deducted for income tax purposes. You should consult with a qualified CPA.

Medical expenses, not compensated for by insurance or otherwise, may be allowed as a deduction. Medical care can include amounts paid for "qualified long-term services" (IRC 213[d]). There are special rules on deducting qualified long-term care costs as medical expenses (IRC 7702B). *Qualified long-term care services* means necessary diagnostic, preventive, therapeutic, curing, treating, mitigating, and rehabilitative services or maintenance, or personal care services required by a chronically ill individual and provided pursuant to a plan of care prescribed by a licensed health care practitioner.

Maintenance or personal care services is defined as care that has as its primary purpose providing needed assistance for a chronically ill individual with his or her disabilities, including protection from threats to health and safety due to severe cognitive impairments.

Chronically ill individual means any individual who has been certified by a licensed health care practitioner as (1) being unable to perform at least two of six specified activities of daily living (eating, toileting, transferring, bathing, dressing, and continence) for a period of at least ninety days due to a loss of functional capacity; (2) having a level of disability similar to the ADL level of disability as determined under regulations prescribed by the secretary of the Treasury in consultation with the secretary of Health and Human Services; or (3) requiring substantial supervision to protect the individual from threats to health and safety due to severe cognitive impairment.

The Internal Revenue Code does not define what a "plan of care" is. For skilled nursing facilities, a written plan of care for each patient is a federal statutory requirement. There is no similar requirement for assisted living facilities (ALFs), but most ALFs do prepare such plans. The plan of care must be prescribed by a licensed health care practitioner, which includes a physician, a registered professional nurse, or a licensed social worker.

Being a resident of an ALF does not automatically qualify an individual as chronically ill for medical expense deduction purposes. If an individual cannot satisfy section 7702B's test, he or she can still deduct under section 213 the percentage of the ALF costs that are attributed to nursing services, but not the percentage attributed to room and board and personal services. The ALF should provide its estimate of the deductible nursing services portion of the bill, and that statement should be attached to Schedule A.

To prospectively secure the tax deduction, you should obtain the opinion of a doctor, nurse, or social worker on the chronic illness issue before admission to a facility and as soon as practical when the family member or friend is providing services. A written plan of care should be prepared by a doctor, nurse, or social worker upon or soon after starting the paid care.

For Medicaid purposes, the payments are considered gratuitous when provided by a family member, unless there is a written contract. Therefore, it is advisable to have a written contract providing for reasonable compensation and specifying the nature of services to be provided.

CHAPTER FIVE

Medicaid Planning

As life expectancies and long-term costs continue to rise, the challenge becomes how to pay for these services. Many people cannot afford to pay $7,200 per month or more for the cost of a nursing home. They may find their life savings wiped out in a matter of months, rather than years.

Fortunately, the Medicaid program is there to help. In fact, in our lifetime, Medicaid has become the long-term care insurance of the middle class. To qualify for Medicaid benefits, however, you must meet certain rules regarding the amount of income and assets that you have. The reason for Medicaid planning is simple, because without planning and advice, many people spend more than they should and jeopardize their family security.

Medicaid is a joint state–federal program. The federal government sets basic requirements, but each state may implement them differently, so the programs vary greatly from state to state. This chapter focuses specifically on Nevada law so that you know what works in Nevada at the time of printing. Medicaid is an extremely complex area, and the rules are constantly changing. It is important to see a qualified certified elder law attorney to go over your situation. Your facts and circumstances can differ from others, and your values and goals may necessitate a different planning strategy.

Applying for Medicaid

The Medicaid application is submitted to the State of Nevada, Department of Human Resources, Welfare Division. Applying for Medicaid entails verification of your financial resources as well as meeting citizenship and residency requirements. You must be a US citizen, lawfully admitted permanent resident, or residing permanently in the United States under color of law.

You will need to provide bank statements and other financial records reflecting your income and assets. This information should be submitted with the application. After review of the initial documents, Medicaid staff frequently sends out a request for additional information, and quick response is required. Make sure you have the documentation you need. Start now by organizing your financial records and saving all your financial documents, such as bank statements and social security award letters.

Exempt Assets and Countable Assets
What Must Be Spent?

To qualify for Medicaid, applicants must pass some fairly strict tests on the amount of assets they can keep. To understand how Medicaid works, we first need to review what are known as exempt and non-exempt (or countable) assets. Exempt assets are those you can keep and still qualify for Medicaid. In general, the following are the primary exempt assets:

- up to $2,000
- home, up to $543,000 in equity (The home must be the principal place of residence.)
- personal belongings and household goods
- one car or truck
- burial spaces and certain related items for applicant and spouse
- up to $1,500 designated as a burial fund for applicant and up to $1,500 as a burial fund for the spouse
- value of life insurance if face value is $1,500 or less (If the face value exceeds $1,500, the cash surrender value of those policies is countable.)

All other assets are generally nonexempt and countable. Basically, all money and property, and any item that can be valued and turned into cash, is a countable asset unless it is an exempt asset. This includes:

- cash, savings accounts, and checking accounts (beyond $2,000)
- certificates of deposit
- stocks, bonds, or mutual funds
- land contracts or mortgages held on real estate sold
- US savings bonds
- individual retirement accounts, pension plans (401[k], 403[b])
- nursing home accounts
- prepaid funeral contracts issued in Nevada
- most trusts
- real estate, other than the residence
- more than one car
- boats or recreational vehicles

Although the Medicaid rules themselves are complicated, it is safe to say that a single person with only exempt assets will qualify for Medicaid.

Joint Accounts

Many people add their children's names to bank accounts and even real property. Medicaid counts the entire value of the asset as available to the applicant unless it can be proved that some or all of the money was contributed by the other person who is on the account.

Transferring Assets

Many people wonder, "Can't I give my assets away?" The answer is, maybe, but only if it is done just right. The law has penalties for people who simply give away their assets to attempt to create Medicaid eligibility. For example, every $7,139 (2014 figure) given away during the five years prior to a Medicaid application creates a one-month period of ineligibility. Even though federal gift tax laws allow you to give away up to $14,000 per year without gift tax consequences, those gifts result in a period of ineligibility for Medicaid. The number used to calculate the ineligibility period changes from time to time.

Certain transfers, such as assets transferred to your spouse or to a blind or disabled child, do not create an ineligibility period. The home may be transferred to a child who has lived there for two years and who cared for the parent, enabling the parent to stay out of a nursing home for at least two years. The home may also be transferred to a sibling with an equity interest who has resided there for at least one year before the other sibling's institutionalization.

Though some families spend virtually all of their savings on nursing-home care, Medicaid often does not require it. Several strategies can be used to protect a family's financial security.

Medicaid Planning for Married Couples

Specific rules protect the spouse who remains at home if the other spouse is going into a nursing home. These rules are called the spousal impoverishment provisions. The intent of the law was to change the eligibility requirements for Medicaid when one spouse needs nursing-home care while the other spouse remains at home. The law recognizes that it makes little sense to impoverish both spouses when only one needs to qualify for Medicaid assistance for nursing-home care.

Under these rules, all the couple's countable assets are added up as of the date the spouse enters the facility. The at-home spouse is allowed to keep one-half of all countable assets up to a maximum of $117,240 (2014 figure). The other half of the countable assets must be "spent down" until $2,000 remains. The at-home spouse is allowed to keep a minimum of $23,448 (2014 figure), even if that is more than half. The amount the at-home spouse can keep is called the community spouse resource allowance (CSRA).

The court may increase the amount of savings the at-home spouse can keep to a sum in excess of one-half of the resources. An experienced elder law attorney can analyze your case and often avoid or reduce the spend-down. Without proper advice, many people spend more money than they have to spend.

Spousal Support

The at-home spouse is entitled to a minimum monthly income of $1,938.75 (2013–14 figure). If the at-home spouse does not have at least $1,938.75 for his or her own income, he or she is allowed to take the income of the nursing-home spouse in the amount necessary to reach $1,938.75. The nursing home spouse's remaining income goes to the nursing home.

Nevada law allows the at-home spouse to seek an increase in the monthly income allowance. The court can increase this allowance up to $2,931 (2014 figure) with a court order. This reduces the necessity for the at-home spouse to dip into savings each month, which would result in gradual impoverishment.

To illustrate, assume the at-home spouse receives $940 per month in income, and her husband receives $1,950 per month in income. Without a court order, she is entitled to the minimum of $1,937.75. Her income is $997.75 less than the monthly income allowance. She will keep her income and receive part of her husband's income to take her total up to $1,937.75 per month. The rest of her husband's income will then go to the nursing home, less his $35 per month personal needs allowance.

With a court order, she may receive up to $2,931 per month. She would receive all the marital income, and none of her husband's income would go to the nursing home.

Case Study: Division of Assets and Spousal Support

Patricia encouraged her parents, Hazel and Harry, to move to Nevada so she could keep a closer eye on them. When they arrived, they purchased a home nearby, and they did well for a while, until Harry had a stroke. Now the family doctor has told Patricia and Hazel that they need to place Harry in a nursing home. Hazel and Harry's assets are as follows:

Savings Account	$49,000
Mutual Funds	$53,000
Checking Account	$ 4,500
Residence (no mortgage)	$120,000

Harry gets a social security check for $1,125 each month; Hazel's check is $600. Her eyes fill with tears as she says, "At over $7,000 to the nursing home every month, our entire life savings will be gone in less than two years." What's more, she is afraid she will not be able to pay her monthly bills, because a neighbor told her that the nursing home will be entitled to all of Harry's social security check.

Although Nevada law allows Hazel to seek an increase in the amount of assets and income she can keep, she must proceed properly. Hazel may be entitled to keep their entire life savings, and Medicaid will pay for Harry's nursing home. She will need to petition a court to increase the assets and income. With proper planning, she can keep everything she and Harry have worked so hard for.

Case Study: Equal Division of Assets

Barbara and Bernard have been married twenty-two years. Barbara suffered a stroke and is getting worse. The couple has accumulated $400,000 in assets, and they have a home. Bernard wants to protect the assets. He says, "I worry about losing everything. I have even thought about getting a divorce. I want to stop worrying. What can I do?"

If Bernard applies through the Welfare Department, they will tell him that he and Barbara have too many assets, and that the most he can keep is $117,240 (2014 figure). But Bernard can save even more, by petitioning the court to divide the assets equally. By doing this, one-half of the assets, or $200,000, is set aside to him and will not have to be used to pay the nursing home for Barbara's care. The couple stays married and can stop worrying about losing all the assets. In addition, there may be other steps available to preserve assets.

Case Study: The Income Cap

Margaret and Sam have been married for forty-one years. After Sam fell and broke his hip, his entire condition rapidly declined. "The doctor says Sam needs long-term care in a nursing home," Margaret says. "The case worker said our income is too high to qualify for Medicaid, and we have to apply through the county after I spend down most of our assets. I don't want to lose all our hard-earned money. I don't know what to do."

Nevada is an income cap state. This means that if the nursing home spouse's income is over the income cap, he or she is not eligible for Medicaid. The monthly income cap amount is $2,163 (2014 figure), and gross figures are used. Medicaid will also add both spouses' income, and if that amount is not more than twice the income cap, the nursing home spouse is not over the income cap.

The couple has $80,000 in savings. Margaret's income from social security is $1,100 per month. Sam's income from social security is $800 per month, and he receives a retirement payout of $2,800 per month. The income is over the income cap. If she proceeds properly, she may be entitled to keep their entire life savings, and Medicaid will pay for the nursing home. She can create an income reduction trust, which is also known as a Miller trust. If this is done, her husband's income is paid out of the trust at a rate that would qualify him for Medicaid. Margaret can then petition the court to increase the assets and income. If she does, Margaret can keep the entire $80,000 in savings as well as the federal maximum in income each month.

Case Study: Financial Gifts to Children

After Harry suffers a paralyzing stroke, Hazel and her daughter, Patricia, need advice. Patricia wants to ensure that her father's medical needs are met, but she also wants to preserve her mother's assets. "Can't Mom just give her money to me as a gift?" she asks. "Can't she give away $14,000 a year? I could keep the money for her so she doesn't lose it when Dad applies for Medicaid."

Patricia has confused federal gift tax law with the issue of transfers and Medicaid eligibility. A gift to a child in this case is actually a transfer, and Medicaid has specific rules about transfers.

At the time Harry applies for Medicaid, the State will "look back" five years to see if any gifts have been made. The State will not let you just give away your money or your property to qualify for Medicaid. Any gifts or transfers for less than fair market value that are uncovered in the look-back period will disqualify Harry from Medicaid for a certain number of months. There are other pitfalls associated with gifting, including tax consequences. Studies have shown that windfall money received by gift, prize, or lawsuit settlement is often gone within three years. In other words, even when the children promise that the money will be available when needed, their own "emergencies" may cause them to spend the money. Furthermore, the money given to your children is subject to attachment by their creditors. We recommend you consult a knowledgeable adviser on how to set a plan that complies with the law and achieves your goal.

Patricia and Hazel decide to do a division of assets and apply for Medicaid for Harry. They consider a written care contract for Patricia's daughter to provide care for Hazel.

The Medicaid Spend-Down

What is a spend-down? This is the amount by which a Medicaid applicant's allowable resources must be reduced to obtain eligibility. The concept applies to both married and single applicants, although married applicants have additional methods of spend-down at their disposal. One method is to pay for the costs of long-term care. Funds can also be used to benefit the applicant or the spouse.

Basic Spend-Down for Married or Single Applicants

Any individual expecting a long nursing-home stay should spend funds on a thorough dental examination and dental work, procuring glasses and other hardware that may be unavailable through Medicaid, purchasing orthopedic shoes, and generally attending to any health-care needs that may be unmet by government benefits.

Expenditures can also be made on items that will improve the quality of life for the resident. Examples include purchase of a television, VCR, stereo, computer, books, tapes, subscriptions, toiletries, or clothing.

Expenditures can also be made to pay off debts; purchase necessary medical supplies and equipment; purchase a burial plot, casket, and marker; or set up a burial account.

Spend-Down for Married Couples

Many spouses are wrongly informed that they must spend down all the resources on nursing home care, but assets can be set aside for the at-home spouse according to the community spouse resource allowance. The amount of the CSRA can be increased by court order.

Exempt property is not counted in determining resources for either spouse for purposes of eligibility. A key concept in spending down to eligibility levels is the conversion of nonexempt resources into exempt resources. This may include:

- purchasing a new residence
- paying down debt on the primary residence
- making necessary repairs and improvements to the home
- purchasing a better vehicle
- purchasing life insurance that does not have cash value

The timing of the spend-down may be critical. Expenditures made before the first institutionalization will reduce the total available resources. That, in turn, could reduce the amount the community spouse is permitted to retain as the CSRA.

Trusts

In Nevada, the use of trusts in Medicaid planning is quite restricted. For Medicaid purposes, the resources in a revocable trust are considered available. An irrevocable trust, with very specific terms, may be created and funded, and after the five-year ineligibility period, the assets will be protected.

A few special trusts are also permitted for Medicaid purposes, but they must be drafted properly. One is a *testamentary trust,* which is created by a will and takes effect upon the death of the person creating the trust. Another exception is a *special needs trust.* This is a trust set up for a disabled person under age sixty-five by a parent, grandparent, legal guardian, or court. The trust must provide for payback to the State upon the death of the beneficiary. If the person is over age sixty-five, the transfer of assets could result in a penalty period. Another exception is a *pooled-income trust,* which is a trust established and managed by a not-for-profit association for the benefit of a person of any age. Transferring some of a person's assets into such a trust can provide for the supplemental needs of the person while that person is on Medicaid.

Will I Lose My Home?

Many people who apply for Medicaid to pay for nursing home care ask, "Will I lose my home?" For many, the home constitutes much or most of their life savings and is usually the greatest asset owned by people facing a long-term care stay. Often, it is the only asset a person has to pass on to his or her children. The home is often the greatest asset not only in terms of monetary value, but also in terms of sentimentality.

Under the Medicaid regulations, the home is an exempt asset. This means that it is not taken into account when calculating eligibility for Medicaid. But in 1993, Congress passed a little-debated law that affects hundreds of thousands of families with a spouse or elderly parent in a nursing home. That law requires states to try to recover the value of Medicaid payments made to nursing home residents. This process is referred to as *Medicaid estate recovery.*

Although the home is an exempt asset for purposes of qualifying for Medicaid, it is not exempt from Medicaid estate recovery. In fact, the home is the asset most frequently sought in this process.

On April 1, 2004, the Nevada Supreme Court ruled on Medicaid estate recovery in the case of *State of Nevada Department of Human Resources v. Estate of Ullmer.* The lower court prohibited the State from placing Medicaid liens against homes of surviving spouses of Medicaid recipients. The Nevada Supreme Court ruled that the State may impose a lien on property in which it has a legitimate interest, subject to certain limitations, before the surviving spouse's death.

The court said that the State "will release the lien upon the surviving spouse's demand for any bona fide transaction, including, but not limited to, selling the property, refinancing the property, and obtaining a reverse mortgage." However, "the State's interest is not extinguished when the deceased recipient's interest in the property is transferred for less than fair market value."

This means that if the surviving spouse wants to sell the house, refinance, or obtain a reverse mortgage, the lien must be lifted, but if the house is gifted to someone, the lien will remain. The court also said that the lien must be limited to the deceased Medicaid recipient's interest in the home. For example, if the husband and wife own the property as joint tenants, then the State can lien only up to a one-half interest in the property.

Review Beneficiary Designations

As a general rule, Medicaid applicants must cash in and spend down all sizeable whole life insurance policies. This is not required for term life insurance policies because they have no cash value. It is important to review both whole life and term policies when applying for Medicaid benefits.

Often people name their spouses as beneficiaries. This can have adverse effects under two circumstances. First, when the insured is the at-home spouse, if he or she predeceases the nursing home spouse, the proceeds of the insurance will go to the surviving nursing home spouse. If the proceeds take the total countable assets over $2,000, the nursing home spouse loses Medicaid eligibility until such insurance proceeds are spent down on his or her care. This concern applies to both whole life and term policies owned by the at-home spouse.

In the other situation, the insured is the nursing home spouse. If the nursing home spouse survives the at-home spouse, the beneficiary clause of the policy will lapse unless an alternate beneficiary has been named. With no alternate beneficiary, the proceeds of the policy will go to the Medicaid recipient's probate estate and be subject to Medicaid estate recovery. In either case, loss of the life insurance proceeds can be prevented by changing the designation of beneficiary. These concerns also apply to other assets with a beneficiary designation.

Planning Strategies

Planning for long-term care costs is complex. You have many routes from which to choose. For those with less than five years to plan, you can still put together the best strategy for your situation. This may include spend-down, converting nonexempt assets into exempt assets, converting nonexempt assets into income, or gifting where exceptions to the rules apply. For married couples, the division of assets and income is another option.

The following are some options for those with more than five years to plan.

Income Trust Fund

This is a fund you create and deposit money into, which you dedicate for paying your long-term care costs. Once you need care, the trustee triggers a lifelong income from the trust that covers the cost of care and is guaranteed by a prearranged contract with an insurer. You cannot outlive the income. Once the trust is properly set up, you must put sufficient money into it, which is why many people do not choose this option. A similar option is to make a lesser deposit to cover you for five years of care. This allows you time to transfer other assets and use the trust to pay for care during the five-year look-back period.

Irrevocable Trust

If there is any circumstance under which payment can be made to or for the benefit of the Medicaid applicant, the part of the trust that could be paid is treated as an available resource. Accordingly, an irrevocable trust must be drafted so that payment cannot be made to the Medicaid applicant. Transferring assets into the irrevocable trust creates a five-year ineligibility period.

Long-Term Care Insurance

To purchase long-term care insurance to cover your care, you must meet health underwriting requirements and pay the premiums. If you purchase a lifetime policy with enough coverage, then you do not need to apply for Medicaid. If you purchase a five-year policy, then you can transfer assets and access the long-term care insurance to pay for care during the five-year look-back period.

People who just sign away financial assets or sign deeds to others are taking huge risks, unless they do some additional smart planning. One significant risk is that the recipient of the assets will spend or lose them, such as through divorce, job loss, bankruptcy, lawsuits, credit card debts, gambling, failed business plans, running off with a new boyfriend or girlfriend, or buying new cars or a house.

Case Study: Irrevocable Trust

Karen has liquid assets of about $250,000, a paid-for home, and a cabin. Ian is her only child. Karen is in fairly good health and is likely to make it five years without needing long-term care; she trusts her son and is willing to make gifts, but she wants to do smart planning. The home and cabin are transferred into an irrevocable trust, starting the five-year penalty period. After five years, the transferred assets are protected. Karen also purchases a product that will provide her with up to $300,000 in long-term care benefits if needed, yet retain a death benefit of $100,000. If care is needed before the five years, the long-term care benefit is accessed.

CHAPTER SIX

Veterans' Benefits

The Department of Veterans Affairs (VA) provides long-term home, community, residential, and nursing home care for veterans. Some of the care is provided in or through the VA's own facilities, and some is contracted with local agencies or facilities.

There is a type of federal pension benefit that may be available to wartime veterans and surviving spouses who have long-term care needs. This benefit is called a *special improved pension* for the veteran and a *death pension* for the single surviving spouse. Both pensions are often referred to as *aid and attendance* benefits, even though that is not the actual name. An understanding of these rules will help position you or your loved one to qualify for these federal benefits.

Another benefit called *compensation* is for veterans and qualifying dependents when the veteran has suffered a disability connected to the service.

Many people do not pursue pension because they think the disability must be service connected. That is not the case for pension benefits. Few people know about the pension benefit for war veterans and their surviving spouses. This chapter is designed to help you understand this underused benefit.

What Is Pension?

Improved pension and death pension are disability income programs available to veterans or to the single surviving spouses of deceased veterans. The veteran had to have served on active duty at least ninety days, with one of those days during a period of war. Two years of active duty is required for those serving in the Gulf War. Service in combat is not required, only that the veteran was in the service during wartime and was discharged other than dishonorably. Charts showing the dates for wartime service are included below.

PERIOD OF WAR	BEGINNING AND ENDING DATES
World War II	December 7, 1941, through December 31, 1946
Korean Conflict	June 27, 1950, through January 31, 1955
Vietnam Era	August 5, 1964, through May 7, 1975; for veterans who served "in country" before August 5, 1964–February 28, 1961 through May 7, 1975
Gulf War	August 2, 1990, through a date to be set by law or presidential proclamation

In order to receive the pension benefit, a veteran household must meet the criteria above as well as meeting an income and asset test and, in most cases, a medical needs test. The VA will deny the application if the net worth is such that part of it could be consumed for the claimant's care. The claimant's countable income cannot exceed the maximum annual pension rate. In computing income, certain items can be deducted from income, including unreimbursed medical expenses paid by a claimant. Many items are included in unreimbursed medical expenses, such as the cost of an assisted living facility, in-home care, adult day care, and nursing home care.

Medical Needs Test

If the veteran is younger than sixty-five, he or she must be permanently and totally disabled. If the veteran is sixty-five or older, there is no disability rating requirement. For single surviving spouses applying for death pension, there is no disability rating requirement. The VA will provide additional income over the basic pension if the claimant meets the requirements for housebound or aid and attendance.

Housebound benefits may be available to a veteran or a single surviving spouse of a veteran who has been determined to be disabled and is essentially confined to the home. Aid and attendance benefits may be available to a veteran or a single surviving spouse of a veteran who meets one of the following conditions: claimant is blind; claimant is living in a nursing home; or claimant has a physical or mental incapacity that requires regular assistance to protect the claimant from daily environmental hazards.

Income Tests

The household income of the veteran or the single surviving spouse cannot exceed the maximum allowable pension rate (MAPR) income for that category of application. Countable income is all income attributable to the claimant, the claimant's spouse, and the claimant's dependent children. The following table lists current MAPR for the year 2013.

STATUS AND MEDICAL RATING	VETERAN	SURVIVING SPOUSE
No medical rating/no dependent	1,038.00	696.00
No medical rating/one dependent	1,360.00	911.00
Housebound rating/no dependent	1,269.00	851.00
Housebound rating/one dependent	1,591.00	1,066.00
Aid and attendance rating/no dependent	1,732.00	1,113.00
Aid and attendance rating/one dependent	2,054.00	1,328.00

For example, a veteran with an aid and attendance medical rating, who is married, cannot make more than $2,054.00 per month from all sources. As another example, a single surviving spouse with a housebound rating cannot make more than $851.00 per month from all sources.

Although most veterans have income that exceeds the permissible family income limits, unreimbursed medical expenses paid by the claimant may be used to reduce the claimant's countable income.

Unreimbursed medical expenses that may reduce income include doctor's fees, dentist's fees, prescription glasses, Medicare premium deductions and co-payments, prescription medications, health insurance premiums, transportation to physician offices, therapy, and funeral expenses. The most beneficial unreimbursed expenses that may reduce countable income are the costs of home health care, adult day care, assisted living facilities, or skilled nursing facilities.

To be able to reduce countable income, a medical rating must be obtained. Certain classes do not require a medical rating to attain pension, but in most cases a medical rating for assistance with two activities of daily living due to disability will be crucial to attaining the benefit. A medical rating allows certain expenses to be annualized and subtracted from future annual income in order to meet the income test. Most veteran households could not obtain pension without this special provision allowing the deduction of annualized unreimbursed medical expenses.

Asset Requirements

The VA considers the net worth of the individual seeking benefits, excluding the value of the person's home, furnishings, and car. The standard for eligibility is whether the person has "sufficient means" to pay for his or her own care. (See M21-1MR, part V, subpart I, chapter 3, section A, 1.d). The net worth of both the veteran and the veteran's spouse are considered when determining eligibility.

No specific dollar amount can be designated as excessive net worth. What constitutes excessive net worth is a question of fact for resolution after considering the facts and circumstances in each case. A number of variables must be taken into consideration when making a net worth determination: (1) income from other sources; (2) family expenses; (3) claimant's life expectancy; and (4) convertibility into cash of the assets involved.

The VA instructs caseworkers to perform an *age analysis* to determine financial need. Under an age analysis, a ninety-eight-year-old person who has $75,000 may not be eligible, whereas seventy-eight-year-old with $75,000 may be considered eligible.

Assets that are not counted include a personal residence, a reasonable amount of land on which it sits, personal property, and automobiles for personal use. Assets that are not readily convertible to cash may be excludable. For married claimants, all assets of both spouses are considered, except in very limited circumstances.

Benefit When Spouse Needs Assistance

If the spouse of the living veteran has a medical need, but the veteran does not have a medical need, limited benefits may be available. The spouse is not permitted to qualify for a rating, but if the spouse meets the medical test, then the expenses can be deducted from income. The veteran is the claimant, not the spouse, and the maximum benefit amount permitted is the basic pension amount. A case example follows.

Richard is eighty-five and lives at home. He still drives, cooks, and plays golf. He is the primary caretaker for his wife, Liz, but the role is becoming increasingly difficult because Liz continues to decline mentally and physically. She is overweight and a fall risk. Therefore, Richard is exploring alternative living arrangements.

He would like to move Liz to an assisted living facility but is afraid he cannot afford it. His son Joe cannot afford to contribute. When Richard was looking at possible assisted living facilities for Liz, he heard about some VA "aid and attendance" benefit. When he called the representative, he was told that he could not get anything from the VA because he was still healthy.

Fortunately, Richard did not give up his quest. Instead, he researched and learned that he could apply for and receive basic pension because:

- he served ninety days during a period of war;
- he received a discharge other than dishonorable;
- he is over age sixty-five (and presumed to be disabled under VA rules);
- his wife meets the medical test, so her assisted living facility expenses can be deducted from income;
- he and his wife's gross monthly income is depleted after deducting recurring, nonreimbursed medical expenses (or would be if she moved into the assisted living facility); and
- they have limited resources.

Richard will not be able to obtain pension with housebound or aid and attendance because he is healthy and not housebound nor is he in need of another person to help him with his daily living activities. Nevertheless, Richard is the VA claimant, is sixty-five years or older, and has limited income and assets that are even more limited when deducting his wife's deductible medical expenses.

Asset Transfers and Tax Implications

Currently, there is no penalty for asset transfers for less than fair market value (gifts) made prior to the application for benefits being submitted. There is a law pending to impose a look-back period. Assets can be gifted to someone who does not live in the household, but they must be completely divested or they will count as net worth. This means outright gifting or transferring into an irrevocable trust with specific qualifying terms.

If there is any possibility that the claimant or the claimant's spouse may require Medicaid to pay for nursing home care in the next five years, then it is not advisable to make gifts, unless other arrangements are made to pay for care during the disqualification period from Medicaid benefits caused by the gifts. Once the look-back period for VA is enacted, then arrangements must be made to pay for care during the disqualification period from VA benefits.

There are tax implications to gifting. Consult a qualified CPA before making gifts. Transfers of ownership for less than fair market value have special meaning from an IRS perspective. Any transfers are clearly gifts for gift tax purposes, and gifts made in excess of $14,000 per year (2013 figure) per individual must be reported on the donor's federal Form 709 gift tax return. The return is required, but there is no tax due unless the total lifetime gifts are greater than the exemption amount.

Assets that are gifted also retain the cost basis of the individual making the gift, but assets that are inherited take on a date-of-death cost basis. From an income tax perspective, it is often a significant disadvantage to have assets gifted rather than being inherited and thus receiving a higher cost basis. Therefore, the possible income tax implications of gifting appreciated assets must be evaluated.

Transferring assets for less than fair market value may not be in the best interest of the claimant. If someone were to report the transfers to Elder Protective Services, the agency may evaluate the situation to determine if exploitation has occurred.

U.S. Series E Bonds that are held for a long period and then liquidated could result in significant income tax due in the year liquidated. This is also true when liquidating life insurance and IRAs.

If the spouse of the claimant is relatively young and healthy, giving away assets is typically not advisable. That spouse then gives up control and autonomy for what is anticipated to be a long time, and serious consideration must be given to weighing the possible benefit against this cost. Keep in mind that a transfer is a completed gift when the claimant no longer has any control over the asset. If the donee dies, the asset will become part of his or her estate, or if that person files bankruptcy, the asset will be used to pay his or her creditors. Specific irrevocable trusts can provide some protection.

If the veteran is receiving military retirement pay, the veteran may also receive pension if the requirements are met. The pension benefit is tax-free income. The IRS generally permits a medical deduction for income tax purposes for nursing home expenses, some assisted living expenses, and some caregiver expenses. Check with your CPA regarding this issue.

Asset Restructuring and Spend-Down

Strategies for restructuring assets or spending down assets to attain eligibility levels may be used in addition to gifting or in lieu of it. Some examples follow.

- Add joint owners to accounts to attain a reduced total value being attributed to the claimant and spouse. Consider the adverse consequences of joint ownership, however, before engaging in this strategy.
- Convert assets into income by annuitizing an annuity, so long as the monthly income generated from the annuity does not increase the income so much that eligibility is lost due to the

excess income. Also, if Medicaid is a possibility, note that it places very specific rules on annuities.

- Pay off debts and make improvements. You can pay off the mortgage, and you can make improvements, repairs, and replacements to the primary place of residence, such as repairing or replacing the roof, painting the house, adding a room, or purchasing new furniture and appliances.
- Convert assets into excluded assets, such as purchasing a new residence; a better vehicle; or life insurance that does not have cash value.
- Purchase items that will improve the quality of life for the claimant or spouse, but that are not considered medical expenses. Examples include purchase of a television, VCR, DVD player, stereo, computer, books, tapes, subscriptions, cell phones, toiletries, or clothing.
- Prepay for funeral arrangements, keeping in mind that burial benefits are available to veterans and their spouses.

Veteran's Spouse Eligibility

For the surviving spouse of an eligible veteran to qualify for death pension, the spouse must have been married to the veteran at the time of the veteran's death, and the spouse cannot have remarried. (There are a few exceptions, such as the surviving spouse remarried and divorced before November 1, 1990.)

Lucy is the widow of a Korean wartime veteran. She was able to stay at home for a while, but then she suffered a stroke, which affected her walking gait, speech, and memory. Lucy's daughter, Maddy, could not supplement her mother's cost of care. The family was desperate, and Maddy did not want her mother to live in a nursing home when an assisted living facility could provide all the care she needed—if only they could afford it.

Maddy had not heard about the benefits available through the VA until her husband's dad applied for them. The additional amount of just over $1,000 per month would help to keep her mother at the assisted living facility so that they did not have to move her to a nursing home. Maddy was overjoyed, because the extra funds per month were all they needed to bridge the shortfall in her income versus the cost of the assisted living facility.

Applying for VA Pension
Supporting Documentation for VA Pension Applications

A key to getting this valuable additional income is knowing what documents and evidence need to be submitted with the claims form. Submitting a substantially complete claim is important to avoid being denied or to having the application process stretch out for a year or more. Benefits are paid retroactively to the first day of the month following the month in which a claim is received by the VA.

Obtaining copies of certain information to present to the VA along with your application is imperative. Documents to include are income statements, social security new benefit amount letters, pension statements, copies of pay checks or stubs, and all other verification of any other type of income, such as interest on securities, rental income, and so forth.

You will also need military discharge papers; your latest bank statements from all financial institutions, including retirement account statements; copies of life insurance policies; your marriage license; and any divorce decrees or death certificates for all prior and current spouses of the claimant and the dependent spouse. In addition, submitting the proper documentation of all medical expenses paid on behalf of the claimant and spouse, including the proper type of physician's statement, is essential.

Appointment of Fiduciary

VA is governed solely by federal law. It requires that the application be signed by the claimant, who is either the veteran or the widow(er). The VA does not recognize powers of attorney or guardianships. If the claimant cannot handle financial affairs, the VA will hold the back benefits due until a VA fiduciary is appointed. If the veteran has a competent spouse, the spouse can receive the money without being appointed fiduciary. Appointment of a VA fiduciary is a separate process and can add substantial delay. If the claimant is incompetent and does not have a spouse, start the fiduciary process immediately.

Death of Claimant

The claim ends with the death of a claimant, but an eligible individual can file for accrued benefits and burial benefits. If a family member had personally paid for expenses related to the last illness of the claimant, they can file a claim for accrued benefits, using Form 21-601. The request for accrued benefits must be filed within one year of the death of the claimant. If the VA actually owed funds to the claimant at the time of the claimant's death, the VA would reimburse only up to what the family member personally paid, not to exceed what was owed to the claimant. If the claimant paid for everything out of his or her own funds and the family did not pay for anything personally, there would be no accrued benefit.

Accredited Agents and Attorneys

As a general rule, only agents and attorneys accredited by the VA may help with the application process. Anyone who is not VA accredited is prohibited from helping someone file a claim even if the person charges no fee. You should select a qualified accredited agent or attorney to assist you.

Notifying VA of Changes

The VA can find that you are qualified to receive benefits but that your benefit is zero or an amount less than the maximum monthly rate, due to not enough unreimbursed out-of-pocket medical expenses. You may be entitled to an increased payment after submitting the proper documentation, usually a Statement in Support of Claim, with appropriate documentation. If circumstances change and you are no longer entitled to the benefit, you need to promptly notify the VA or you could owe a refund.

Information submitted, including income information, is subject to verification through computer-matching programs with other agencies. If you receive distributions from an annuity or other source, whether monthly or otherwise, this income must be reported to the VA. Failure to report this information could result in a demand for overpayment.

You should keep all financial and medical records that are applicable to your initial application for at least seven years.

Other VA Benefits

If your loved one is a veteran, he or she may be eligible to reside in the veteran's facility in Boulder City. The current rate for the veteran is about half of what it would cost in other skilled nursing facilities. Other VA benefits may be available to the veteran or dependent, such as health care benefits. To receive health care benefits, the veteran must "enter the system." To do so, the veteran must complete and file a VA Form 10-10EZ—Application for Medical Benefits (Enrollment Form). Contact the Veterans Benefits Administration for more information.

Case Study: Single Veteran

Patricia and Jim finally got Jim's dad, George, to a doctor. George's doctor says he needs to move to an assisted living facility to protect himself from the hazards of daily living and to get help with bathing, dressing, and eating. His income from social security is $1,000, and his assets total $25,000. The assisted living facility charges a monthly fee of $2,700. Subtracting the cost of the assisted living facility from George's income yields a deficit of $1,700 per month. George is entitled to the maximum payment for a veteran with no dependents.

A medical need for assistance or supervision due to disability is in most cases crucial to getting the pension benefit. A medical rating or a medical need for this disability care allows certain medical expenses to be annualized and subtracted from future annual income in order to meet the income test. Most veteran households could not receive the pension benefit without this special provision allowing the deduction of annualized medical expenses associated with disability.

If a potential claimant were to call a local regional office, the caller may be told there is no benefit if his or her household income exceeds the MAPR for that particular type of application category. In many cases, this is simply not accurate. Keep in mind, however, that some local regional offices are aware of the special medical deduction and may not discourage callers in cases such as these.

Household income can be reduced to meet the pension income test under the special conditions we have mentioned above. This allows households earning $2,000 to $6,000 or more a month to qualify, even though their current nonadjusted income does not meet the income test.

This special provision for annualizing and deducting medical costs associated with a rating also applies to home care costs. Home care costs can include the costs of professional aides or money paid to members of the family (not including the spouse), friends, or people hired independently to provide care in the home.

Deductibility of Family Caregiver Payments

Payments to a family caregiver may be considered unreimbursed medical expenses for VA purposes if the situation meets several requirements. First, the caregiver cannot be the spouse. Second, the care needs to be prescribed by a physician on the proper form. Without a doctor stating the need, the VA is not likely to accept any care expense as an unreimbursed medical expense, regardless of the provider.

Third, the claimant must write a check each month to the caregiver. We recommend keeping documented proof of the exchange for at least five years. Note that the caregiver may have a personal tax liability.

Fourth, the care must be adequately documented to meet VA rules. We recommend a caregiver contract and a caregiver affidavit to meet these requirements. If the fees for an in-home attendant are an allow-able expense, receipts or other documentation of this expense are required. Documentation includes a receipt bill, statement on the pro-vider's letterhead, computer summary, ledger, or bank statement. The evidence submitted must include the amount paid, the date payment was made, the purpose of the payment (the nature of the product or service provided), the name of the person to or for whom the product or service was provided, and identification of the provider to whom pay-ment was made. (See M21-1MR, part V, subpart i, chapter 3, section D).

Some people ask, "Why couldn't the veteran pay the caregiver and then the caregiver pay the veteran's rent?" There would need to be a caregiver affidavit for care given by the caregiver to the claimant and a renter's agreement showing that the payment paid to the claimant is indeed rent. Paying rent may not work because the claimant would have additional income in the form of rent to declare to the VA.

Sometimes the family wants to hire a family member to provide the same care as a professional. The three requirements above must be met. The VA should be notified with proper documentation. Otherwise, an overpayment could be created. A new physician's affidavit is not required if the first one was done correctly, stating the need for care.

Case Study: Aid and Attendance

Sam is in a nursing home after falling and breaking his hip. His wife, Margaret, obtained a division of assets and Medicaid eligibility to pay for her husband's care in the nursing home. Sam slowly improved over time, and both he and Margaret want him to come home. However, Sam still needs assistance, and Margaret is too frail to provide him with the help he needs at home.

There is a lovely assisted living facility just around the corner from their house, and Margaret wants to move her husband there, even though his care is being paid for by Medicaid in the nursing home. Mar-garet's income from social security is $1,100 per month. Sam's income from social security is $800 per month, and he receives a retirement payment of $2,800 per month. Their income is too high to qualify for the home and community–based waiver program. Sam is a veteran of World War II and could be eligible for aid and attendance to help pay the monthly fee at the assisted living facility, which is about $3,900. After deducting the cost of care from their income, Sam can qualify for the aid and attendance benefit and move to the assisted living facility.

CHAPTER SEVEN

Protecting Legal Rights

Whether you or your loved one is attempting to continue living independently or is in a long-term care facility, being prepared with necessary legal documents and understanding and protecting your legal rights are all important. In this chapter, we discuss the legal documents for health care decision making, how you can protect yourself with advance directives, and how these documents can help you make decisions on behalf of others. We also discuss patient's rights, durable power of attorney for financial matters, elder exploitation, and guardianship.

Advance Directives

An advance directive is a document that allows you to state your choices for health care or to name someone to make those choices for you should you become unable to do so. Under Nevada law, advance directives include the living will, the durable power of attorney for health care, the do-not-resuscitate order, and the physician order for life-sustaining treatment.

Becoming involved in your loved one's medical care is important for developing a strategy to keep him or her living independently as long as possible. The time may come when you must take charge of your loved one's medical care due to a sudden crisis situation. If he or she is already in crisis and has not previously given you durable power of attorney for health care, you may need to look into becoming a guardian. This is one reason it is important to plan ahead and execute advance directives, while your loved one has capacity.

Advance directives and end-of-life choices are essential to a cohesive plan of care. Intellectually we understand that we are mortal beings, but people do not want to think about their own death or the death of a beloved. When we do talk about this issue, we soon discover that most folks are not necessarily afraid of death, but are afraid of the process of dying. People often fear that signing a health care directive means that they have lost their power to change their minds about how they want to be treated.

Your loved ones need to know what you want before you can no longer express those wishes. Health care professionals need to know that your loved ones speak for you with one voice and that this voice is yours. In addition to helping your loved ones, documenting your choices will be a tremendous help for those medical professionals entrusted with your care.

Living Wills

A living will is a written declaration stating your wishes regarding the use of life-prolonging medical treatment. Nevada law gives you the option of completing two kinds of living wills, or *declarations*. First is a declaration in which you direct your attending physician to withhold or withdraw life-sustaining treatment. Second is a declaration appointing another person to make the decision for you about withholding life-sustaining treatment.

Any person age eighteen or older and of sound mind may execute a living will. The living will must be signed by the person completing it and must be witnessed by two other persons. Under Nevada law, you can revoke your living will at any time and in any manner, without regard to your mental or physical condition at the time of revocation. A revocation is effective when it is communicated to your attending physician or other health care provider. Once communicated, the physician is required to put the revocation in your record.

Durable Power of Attorney for Health Care

With a durable power of attorney for health care, you name the person you want to make medical decisions for you only if you become incapacitated and are unable to make your own decisions. Unlike a living will, a durable power of attorney for health care can be used for any incapacity. The term *durable* means that the document is still effective when the person who executed it becomes incapacitated. You also state your wishes regarding the type of treatment you want or do not want.

Any person age eighteen or older and of sound mind may execute a durable power of attorney for health care. The durable power of attorney for health care must be signed and acknowledged by a notary public or signed by two qualified witnesses. Neither of the witnesses can be a health care provider, an employee of a health care provider or facility, an operator of a health care facility, or the person you name as attorney-in-fact. One of the witnesses must be unrelated to you by blood, marriage, or adoption, and not be entitled to any part of your estate. You may not appoint as your health care agent a health care provider or employee, or a health facility operator or employee, unless the person is your spouse, guardian, or next of kin.

Under Nevada law, a certification of competency must be attached to the durable power of attorney for health care if the person executing the power of attorney resides in a hospital, residential facility for groups (this includes group homes and assisted living facilities), a nursing home, or a home for individual residential care. The certification must be from a physician, psychologist, or psychiatrist. If the certification of competency is not attached to the power of attorney for health care executed in Nevada, then it is not valid.

Under Nevada law, a durable power of attorney for health care will remain in effect indefinitely, unless you revoke it or specifically provide in the document that you wish it to terminate on an earlier date. If a guardian is later appointed for you, the power of attorney for health care is revoked, but the guardian still must follow your known wishes.

Do-Not-Resuscitate Orders

A do-not-resuscitate (DNR) order is an order entered by a physician that you not be resuscitated. The term *do not resuscitate* is a terrifying one, and several hospices and hospitals nationwide have begun to use the phrase "allow a natural death" in its place. To experience a natural death changes the dynamic from refusal to permission and may make the decision easier to understand and process.

For now, in Nevada, DNR is the name of the order. While you are in a health care facility, the DNR order will apply as long as your medical record with the DNR order documented is available.

Emergency personnel will not recognize a living will or durable power of attorney for health. They are required by law to resuscitate in the event of cardiac or respiratory arrest unless presented with a DNR identification card issued in Nevada or a DNR bracelet issued by another state. If emergency personnel are presented with a valid DNR card, they will withhold life-resuscitating treatment such as CPR, defibrillation, intubation, ventilator assistance, and cardiac resuscitation drugs. If you have a valid DNR identification card, you will receive all appropriate care that would normally be provided, up until such time as you develop cardiac or respiratory arrest. Such care includes oxygen, pain medication, and positioning for comfort.

If you are at home or in an assisted living facility and do not want to be resuscitated, you should submit a DNR Identification Application to the health district in the appropriate county. The application must be signed by a physician certifying that you have a terminal condition. You or your agent must also sign the application, stating that you do not wish to receive life-resuscitating treatment. After receipt of the signed application, the health district will then issue a salmon-colored DNR identification card. To obtain a DNR application, call the Alzheimer's Association or the appropriate health district.

Physician Order for Life-Sustaining Treatment

A physician order for life-sustaining treatment (POLST) form states what kind of medical treatment you want toward the end of your life. Printed on bright paper and signed by both you and a doctor, POLST helps give you more control over your end-of-life care. The POLST form gives direction to a health care provider regarding the use of emergency care and life-sustaining treatment. It is intended to be honored by any provider of health care who treats you in any setting, including your home or a health care facility, or even at the scene of a medical emergency.

A physician is required to explain to you the existence and availability of the POLST form, the features of the POLST form, and the difference between a POLST form and the other types of advance directives. This is to occur if the physician diagnoses you with a terminal condition, if the physician determines you have a life expectancy of less than five years, or at your request. At your request, the physician must complete the POLST form based on your preferences and medical indications. The POLST form is valid upon execution by a physician and you, while competent. If you are no longer competent, then the POLST form can be signed by your representative, which means your legal guardian, the person you designated in your living will, or the person you designated in your durable power of attorney for health care.

A POLST form may be revoked at any time and in any manner by you, if competent, or by your representative, if you are not competent. The health care provider must make the revocation a part of your medical record. A physician may evaluate you and, based on the evaluation, may recommend new orders consistent with the most current health information.

If the POLST form conflicts with any of your other advance directives, the declaration, direction, or order set forth in the document executed most recently is valid, and any other declarations, directions, or orders that do not conflict remain valid. If your POLST form sets forth an order to provide life-resuscitating treatment and you also have a

DNR identification, a health care provider shall not provide life-resuscitating treatment if the DNR identification is with you when the need for life-resuscitating treatment arises.

Substituted Judgment

If you are no longer competent, and do not have an advance directive, surrogate decision makers are authorized by statute to decide issues regarding life-sustaining treatment. The statute lists who may make the decision in the following order of priority: spouse or registered domestic partner, majority of adult children, parents, majority of siblings, or nearest other adult relative by blood or adoption.

A Nevada Supreme Court case, *Estate of Maxey v. Darden,* 187 P.3d 144 (Nev. 2008), addressed multiple sections of Nevada's Uniform Act on Rights of the Terminally Ill, codified in NRS 449.535 through 449.690. Avis Maxey, who was seventy-two years old, ingested approximately two hundred prescription pills in an apparent suicide attempt. Her ex-husband, Theodore, with whom she resided, delayed calling an ambulance because he believed she wanted to kill herself. When the paramedics arrived, they nonetheless attempted to resuscitate Avis. At the hospital, Theodore signed papers listing Avis as a class III patient, meaning her treatment would be limited to comfort care without prolonging her life. A doctor signed the order and later extubated Avis on Theodore's request.

Avis was given an oxygen mask, but that was removed ten minutes later "per husband's request." Over the next three hours, Avis's respirations decreased. The shift changed, and a different doctor ordered a morphine drip. Avis died soon thereafter, approximately four hours and twenty minutes after admission to the hospital. Later, the family filed a malpractice action.

The Uniform Act on Rights of the Terminally Ill permits an attending physician to withhold or withdraw life-sustaining treatment from a terminally ill patient based on three methods: (1) declaration from the patient, (2) declaration from the patient's designee, or (3) in the absence of either declaration, surrogate consent from certain family members.

Avis had not executed a declaration concerning her end-of-life wishes and had not designated a health care decision maker. Therefore, the case turned on whether her doctor received valid surrogate consent before withholding treatment. Although Theodore was the ex-husband and not entitled to give consent under the act, he presented as her husband, and the emergency room doctor was unable to ascertain his status as ex-husband.

The surrogate must consent in writing to withdrawing or withholding life-sustaining treatment, "attested by two witnesses." Only the emergency room doctor witnessed the consent, and the nurse made chart notes. There was an issue of fact as to whether the chart notes would be considered a proper attestation by a second witness. This case illustrates the importance of executing advance directives and executing them properly.

Living Will Registry

Once you have your advance directives in place, you may have them stored electronically in the Nevada Living Will Lockbox through the Secretary of State's Office. The lockbox is a secure web-based registry that was authorized by the 2007 Nevada legislature. The lockbox allows authorized health care providers to have immediate access to your medical directives. You may also provide loved ones access to your medical directives by giving them your password.

The Nevada Secretary of State encourages the use of Nevada's Living Will Lockbox, stating:

> I know you fully understand the function and value of advance directives, and realize they are essentially ineffective if they are not readily available when critical health care decisions must be made. The Living Will Lockbox is the best way to securely store advance health care directives while still ensuring those important documents are readily available to health care providers at times of crisis. Use of the Living Will Lockbox is

free to all Nevadans and registering is very simple. By visiting www.livingwilllockbox.com, you can download the registration forms and send the completed forms and advance directives to be filed with the Living Will Lockbox to the Nevada Secretary of State. Once registered, you will receive a wallet card with your password for accessing your advance directives. Changes to the documents may be made at any time through a simple procedure similar to the registration process.

HIPAA

HIPAA stands for the Health Insurance Portability and Accountability Act, which establishes national standards for the protection of health information. HIPAA privacy rules limit the circumstances in which an individual's protected health information may be used or disclosed. This means that a doctor may not talk to you about your loved one's condition unless you have specific authority. The agent named in the durable power of attorney for health care may be legally authorized to obtain this information, making it vital that the durable power of attorney for health care be executed to facilitate the eldercare plan. Your loved one can also execute a specific HIPAA authorization that will give the people named in the authorization the authority to obtain medical information. His or her physicians, hospital, or nursing home can give you the HIPAA form to execute.

Improving the Effectiveness of Advance Directives

Do not just rely on checking a few boxes on an advance directive form. Pose the following questions: At what point in a person's health does it make sense not to extend all the medical options? Does your mother want to have all the bells and whistles used if she has severe dementia? How would your husband feel about prolonging his life if he will be in unending pain and disability with no hope to improve?

The more specific you can be, the less stress your loved ones will experience while struggling to decipher exactly what you meant. Specificity generally leads to fewer arguments among family members about necessary medical decisions in a time of crises. During any period of your loved one's incapacity, the health care agent should expect to be actively involved in decision making. Care providers need to be consulted, second opinions considered, and the burdens and benefits of proposed treatments balanced.

The wishes of the loved one are paramount, and Nevada law requires the agent to follow the known wishes of the principal. This means that agents first consider not what they think is best but the expressed direction of the principal from the document itself. When the agent knows that the principal would refuse treatment, and the refusal is likely to result in death, the agent may not choose to allow treatment despite the principal's wishes.

No matter what age, we all need to consider the importance of letting loved ones know exactly what we want should a terminal illness or mental incapacity make us unable to speak for ourselves.

Pain Management

Severe pain or other distressing symptoms are not something you should accept as a "normal" part of living with a serious illness. Physicians are required to provide treatment that is necessary for comfort or to alleviate pain.

Hospice programs are experienced in providing palliative care. Hospice care is an interdisciplinary approach that provides comfort, rather than curative, care to those with a life-limiting illness. It covers pain control and counseling, including bereavement counseling for caregivers and family.

The term *palliative care* refers to more than just pain management. It concentrates on helping people be comfortable by looking after their medical, emotional, social, and spiritual needs. Hospice and other palliative care providers have special training to provide this kind of care. Hospitals also provide palliative care. The goals of palliative care are to improve the quality of a seriously ill person's life and to support the person and his or her family during and after treatment. Hospice may be provided at home, in nursing homes, in hospitals, or in special inpatient units.

Patient's Rights

Patient's rights come in various forms and from multiple sources. Nevada has passed laws creating patient's rights, and federal law also provides patient's rights. Patients in a facility that receives Medicare or Medicaid payments have rights under federal law. A highlight of some federal patient's rights follows.

Right to Autonomy, Dignity, and Respect

Residents have the right to make their own schedule and choose which activities they attend, as long as it is not adverse to their care plan. In making their own schedule, residents have the right to decide what time they wake up in the morning, what time they eat their meals, and what time they go to bed at night.

Right to Manage Own Finances

Nursing home residents have the right to make their own financial and medical decisions, including the right to check out of the nursing home unless the court has appointed a guardian to make those decisions.

Right to Participate in Plan of Care

Residents have the right to full participation in their health care planning, including the right to refuse services and the right to refuse medical treatment. Residents have the right to participate in their own care-plan meetings and invite whom they want to attend.

Right to Be Free from Abuse and Restraints

Residents have the right to be free from physical, sexual, verbal, and mental abuse. Residents have the right to be free from unnecessary physical or chemical restraints, and such restraints are not to be used for disciplinary measures, nor may they be used for staff convenience.

Right to Confidentiality

All information regarding personal, financial, medical, and social affairs is privileged and is to be kept confidential.

Right to Be Fully Informed

Residents have the right to be informed of their rights, and to be informed of services offered and charges for those services, including those not covered by the facility's daily rate. Residents have the right to be informed of their medical condition and treatment plan. Residents have the right to receive notice of changes concerning their treatment.

Right to Choose One's Own Physician

Residents must be able to choose their own doctor and pharmacy.

Right to Voice Grievances

Every nursing home must have a system to address concerns relating to residents' treatment or care, and post pertinent information regarding advocacy for patients. Residents have the right to prompt efforts for resolution by the nursing home, and to be free from retaliation.

Right to Privacy

Residents have the right to privacy, including meeting privately with any visitors; sending and receiving private, unopened mail; and making private telephone calls.

Right Against Unlawful Discharge or Transfer

A nursing facility may discharge a resident only for specific reasons and with a thirty-day written notice.

Power of Attorney for Finances

A power of attorney is a legal document in which one person (the principal) authorizes another (the agent) to act on his or her behalf. The principal specifies what authority the agent has and when the document is effective. You can name more than one agent and should consider naming successor agents.

Nevada has adopted the Uniform Power of Attorney Act. Unless the power of attorney specifically states otherwise, various powers and limitations are as provided by statute. For example, unless the power of attorney provides otherwise, co-agents may act independently.

The power of attorney is effective when executed unless the principal provides that the power of attorney become effective at a future date or upon the occurrence of a future event. Usually, the specified event is the incapacity of the principal, who can specify the persons authorized to determine incapacity.

A certification of competency must be attached to the power of attorney for finances if the person executing the power of attorney resides in a hospital, residential facility for groups (including group homes and assisted living facilities), nursing home, or home for individual residential care. The certification must be from a physician, psychologist, or psychiatrist. If the certification of competency is not attached to the power of attorney for assets executed in Nevada, then the power of attorney is not valid.

Banks and other institutions often seek to limit powers of attorneys. Under the Uniform Power of Attorney Act, an entity or person must accept an acknowledged (notarized) power of attorney, or request that the agent provide a certification or an opinion of counsel. Upon receipt of the certification or opinion of counsel, the institution or person must accept the power of attorney within five business days, with some exceptions. One exception is knowledge that a report has been made that the principal may be subject to abuse, neglect, exploitation, or isolation by the agent or a person acting for or with the agent. Failing to comply with these procedures may subject the person who is presented with the power of attorney to pay attorney's fees.

An agent must act in accordance with the principal's reasonable expectations to the extent actually known by the agent and, otherwise, in the principal's best interest. The agent must act in good faith and only within the scope of authority granted in the power of attorney.

These requirements cannot be waived, even if the power of attorney says otherwise.

Unless the power of attorney provides otherwise, an agent has the following obligations: (1) act loyally for the principal's benefit; (2) act so as not to create a conflict of interest; (3) act with care, competence and diligence ordinarily exercised by agents; (4) keep a record of all receipts, disbursements, and transactions made on behalf of the principal; (5) cooperate with a person that has authority to make health care decisions; and (6) attempt to preserve the principal's estate plan. Interested parties may petition a court to review the agent's conduct. An agent who violates the statute is liable to the principal for the amount required to restore the value of the property to what it would have been had the violation not occurred.

A durable power of attorney for assets terminates when the principal dies, when the principal revokes the power of attorney or the agent's authority, or when the power of attorney provides that it terminates. If a court appoints a guardian of the estate, the power of attorney for assets is terminated unless the guardianship court specifically permits the power of attorney to remain valid. A power of attorney for assets also terminates if the agent dies, becomes incapacitated, or resigns and there is no successor agent named in the power of attorney. To avoid having no one with authority to act, consider naming trustworthy successor agents.

Elder Abuse and Exploitation

As our parents and other loved ones age, they may become lonely and vulnerable to scams or exploitation. Our office frequently hears about elderly widows who become victims of con artists wanting them to wire money to claim a "prize" the women allegedly won. Almost half of substantiated cases involved individuals who were unable to care for themselves; many are confused or suffering from some degree of depression.

The best way to avoid problems later on is to plan ahead. Ideally, your loved one should have an estate plan in place that includes powers of attorney for health care and for finances as well as a revocable living trust that specifies who will manage the finances and under what circumstances. Additionally, your loved one should maintain updated lists of income and assets.

You can take various steps to protect your elders from being taken advantage of by con artists, high-pressure salespeople, and even legitimate groups.

- Put your loved one on do-not-call lists. Most telemarketers will stop calling once a number has been on the National Do Not Call Registry for thirty-one days. You can register home and cell phone numbers for free at donotcall.gov or by calling 888-382-1222.

- Monitor the mail. Tell your loved one that you have heard about scams targeting seniors and that you want to help protect them. If you live in the same town, ask him or her to collect the mail during the week so that you can go through it and write checks together. Otherwise, ask a trusted person to help weed out questionable mail and requests for money.

- Monitor accounts. Look at bank and credit card statements with your loved one and ask about questionable payments. If your loved one is willing, consider becoming a power of attorney on the account so that you can receive bank statements or set up online banking to monitor activity. You may also want to get copies of his or her credit reports at www.annualcreditreport.com to make sure your loved one is not a victim of identity theft.

- Limit access to cash and credit. If your loved one has dementia, the above steps will probably not be enough to protect him or her from scams, particularly as the disease progresses. You can start by setting up automatic payments for regular bills to reduce the number of checks that need to be written. If you have access to your loved one's checking account, limit the amount of money in it by regularly transferring funds to a savings or money-market account. Consider a secured credit card, which allows a deposit that becomes the credit limit, and take away the other cards. Consider giving your loved one a cash allowance.

If your loved one is not willing to take these steps or otherwise protect him- or herself, consider a referral to the appropriate agency, such as Elder Protective Services. In some situations, a guardianship may be warranted. If your loved one is exploited by a family member, it can be difficult to distinguish a transfer of assets made with consent from an exploitative transaction resulting from undue influence, duress, fraud, coercion, or lack of informed consent.

Guardianship

If your loved one is incapacitated and cannot make decisions, then legal documents cannot be executed. In this situation, you may have to go to court to appoint a legal guardian to act on his or her behalf.

Under Nevada law, the court will appoint a general guardian if the proposed ward is "incompetent," or a special guardian if the person is of "limited capacity." *Incompetent* means "an adult person who, by reason of mental illness, mental deficiency, disease, weakness of mind or any other cause, is unable, without assistance, properly to manage and take care of himself or his property, or both. The term includes a mentally incapacitated person" (NRS 159.019). A person is of *limited capacity* if he or she is not a minor and "is able to make independently some but not all of the decisions necessary for the person's own care and the management of the person's property" (NRS 159.022).

To obtain a guardianship, recent medical documentation must support the need for one. Alternatively, a public agency charged with investigations may support the need for guardianship. Nevada also permits voluntary guardianships when the proposed ward consents to one.

Under Nevada law, one of the guardians must be a Nevada resident. If you reside outside Nevada, professional guardians may serve along with family members. If someone has no family, or no one willing to serve, a professional guardian may serve alone.

If your loved one retains some degree of orientation and capability, then a court proceeding can be emotionally devastating. A special guardianship is often a way to provide help and protection without a finding of incompetency. Although general guardianship is a serious step, sometimes it is the only choice to help your loved one. Again, it is important to plan early to avoid the need for guardianship proceedings.

Think about Patricia. She has had a lot on her plate, dealing with her parents and Jim's father, George. For some time, she noticed signs that her husband was not the same and was becoming more forgetful. She finally took him to a doctor, and he was diagnosed with Alzheimer's disease, just as George had been. Jim's condition got worse. He could no longer handle his own affairs, much less help with his father's needs. George had executed a power of attorney for health care and a power of attorney for finances, but he had made a serious error. He had named his only son, Jim, as the agent and no alternate agent. Jim lost his capacity, so he can no longer serve as agent under his father's power of attorney. George lacks the capacity to execute a new power of attorney. Patricia now must contend with petitioning the court to become George's guardian. If she had been named as an alternate on George's documents, this could have been avoided.

CHAPTER EIGHT

The Affordable Care Act in Nevada

The Patient Protection and Affordable Care Act (ACA) of 2010, as amended, changes the nation's health care system. This chapter provides an overview of what it will mean for you and your loved ones, as well as how it is being implemented in Nevada.

Overview of the ACA

The stated purposes of the ACA were primarily to insure more Americans, to control health care costs, and to add more consumer benefits and protections. In its effort to decrease the number of uninsured, the ACA has the individual mandate, which makes it a requirement for every American to get health insurance or pay a fine. The ACA then offers three ways to help: the expansion of Medicaid, the creation of health insurance exchanges, and the addition of financial incentives for small businesses.

After the ACA was enacted in 2010, twenty-six state governments mounted a legal challenge to the law, and Nevada was one of those states. In June 2012, the Supreme Court of the United States upheld the ACA's individual mandate provision under the federal government's power to impose taxes on citizens. But the Supreme Court also ruled that the federal government could not force individual states to expand Medicaid coverage within their borders against their will. The federal government is encouraging states to expand Medicaid by covering almost all the cost of those newly eligible from 2014 to 2020. Nevada has chosen the Medicaid expansion.

Medicaid will be expanded to provide health insurance for more low-income Nevadans by making it available to those with incomes up to 138 percent of federal poverty level. The ACA states that Medicaid is to be increased up to 133 percent of federal poverty level, but there is a 5 percent income disregard, which effectively makes it 138 percent. The ACA has no effect on institutional Medicaid in Nevada, which is the Medicaid program for the aged, blind, and disabled to pay for the cost of long-term care.

Many people eligible under the old rules did not participate. More of these people are likely to sign up to avoid the penalty. The financial burden for Nevada will be heavier because the federal government will pay for those previously eligible under the old formula, which covers about 57 percent of their cost on average.

In 2010, about 85 percent of Americans had health insurance, with 48 percent through their employers, 15 percent from Medicare, 13 percent from Medicaid, and 9 percent buying individual health care coverage. Most of the remaining 15 percent were uninsured, with a big portion of this group being illegal aliens. Among those citizens who were uninsured, many were adults in good health, while others were the medically uninsurable who were not eligible for Medicare or Medicaid. The ACA is designed to insure this last group.

After the ACA goes into full operation, those who remain uninsured will primarily be illegal aliens, who will remain ineligible for Medicaid and will not be allowed to buy insurance through the exchanges. The others who remain uninsured will be those people who refuse to comply with the individual mandate.

Exploding medical costs are a big and growing problem, not only making it difficult to afford health insurance, but also increasing the costs to run Medicare and Medicaid. The ACA attempts to reduce medical costs mainly by encouraging a movement away from the current fee-for-service system.

There are significant consumer protections under the ACA. For example, insurance plans can no longer impose an annual limit or a lifetime limit on a policyholder's benefits. Insurance companies can no longer refuse to extend coverage because of a pre-existing health condition or charge a higher premium to people who are older or have a chronic disease.

The ACA only applies to employers with more than fifty full-time employees. Employers with more than fifty full-time employees must offer a health insurance package for employees that meets the federal essential health benefits and does not cost the employees more than 9.5 percent of their annual salary. Potential penalties will be assessed to employers with more than fifty full-time employees. The penalty will be $3,000 per employee, with a cap. More than 1,500 waivers have been granted to certain companies and unions, allowing noncompliance with the requirements of the ACA.

Silver State Health Insurance Exchange

The ACA requires that each state have a health insurance exchange. States may create and run their own, partner with other states, or let the federal government run their exchange. Nevada received approval from the U.S. Department of Health and Human Services to run its own exchange, which is called the Silver State Health Insurance Exchange. While Nevada mounted its challenge against the ACA, it also prepared to run its own exchange in the event the ACA was upheld, in order to protect Nevadans and design an exchange in consideration of our economy and demographics. Nevada's exchange is one of the best and its readiness was timely.

Multiple health insurance plans are housed on the exchange, where consumers can compare plans. Plans sold through the exchange by different insurance companies must contain identical levels of benefits at specific tiers of coverage so that consumers can make accurate comparisons between the plans. Each plan must cover essential health benefits.

You can access the exchange directly through the Internet, over the phone, or at government offices. If you call or stop by an office, an exchange employee will put all information directly into the Internet portal for the exchange.

Nevadans may purchase health insurance on the exchange, but

illegal aliens are excluded. The exchange does not offer enrollment in Medicare. It offers qualified health plans for people age sixty-four or under. Those on Medicaid also do not need to purchase health insurance on the exchange. If you have insurance through your employer, you do not need to purchase through the exchange, but the exchange is open to workers whose employers offer them health insurance that does not cover at least 60 percent of their medical costs, or if the employee's share of premiums exceeds 9.5 percent of his or her wages.

Insurance carriers that offer qualified health plans on the exchange offer the same product outside the exchange. The exchange is the only place where you can receive premium assistance in the form of an advance premium tax credit or cost-sharing reductions. The advance premium tax credit is not available if you earn more than 400 percent of poverty level, and the cost-sharing reduction is not available if you earn more than 250 percent of poverty level.

If an employer provides affordable minimum essential coverage for its employees, the employees are not eligible for tax credits on the individual exchange. During the enrollment process, employees must attest that they do not have access to affordable minimum essential coverage, and they must list their employer. The exchange will contact employer to verify that the employee does not have access to minimum essential coverage. Employers will not be penalized for an employee who does not elect to participate in an employer-sponsored health insurance plan that is affordable and meets the minimum essential coverage.

The exchange has four standardized plans: bronze, silver, gold, and platinum. Each is required to include essential health benefits. After the minimum level of benefits is met, the tiers of coverage differ based on the amount of financial coverage the plans offer, with bronze covering 60 percent of medical costs on average, silver at 70 percent, gold at 80 percent, and platinum at 90 percent.

SHOP Exchange

Under the ACA, small businesses can purchase insurance through a SHOP exchange, which is officially called the Small Business Health

Option Program. In Nevada, the Silver State Health Insurance Exchange administers SHOP. In Nevada, it is available for businesses with up to fifty employees in 2014, increasing to up to one hundred employees in 2016. Employees log on and choose a coverage plan from the plans that the employer selected. Employers will receive one easy-to-read bill from the exchange for all their employees.

In 2017, states may open the SHOP exchange to large employers if they choose. Unless that occurs, the only time the exchange would come into play for a large business is if the large business decides to stop offering health insurance, pay the fine, and send the employees to the individual exchange for coverage.

How the ACA Affects Medicare

Medicare is one of the most important components of the health care system, providing coverage for citizens age sixty-five and over. ACA includes one significant improvement to Medicare but also makes Medicare a target for spending cuts. Under the ACA, the infamous "doughnut hole" in Medicare's prescription drug coverage will be slowly phased out by 2020. By 2020, for brand-name drugs, the pharmacy industry will cover 50 percent, Medicare recipients will cover 25 percent, and the federal government will provide a subsidy. For generic drugs, Medicare recipients will pay 25 percent, and the federal government will provide a subsidy for the rest. Means testing will expand under Medicare, so that individuals with an income of $85,000 or higher and couples with an income of $170,000 or higher will receive a reduced subsidy, which will increase the price they pay for their prescriptions.

Seniors are wondering who is going to pay for the ACA. According to the Congressional Budget Office, hundreds of billions of dollars in funding for ACA will be generated by cuts in Medicare's budget over the next decade. The biggest spending cuts will come in reducing the number of plans available, the benefits in the Medicare Advantage program, and the payment rates to doctors who care for Medicare patients. Perhaps of more concern for seniors is the presidential commission called the Independent Payment Advisory Board. This board will be given signif-

icant power to cut Medicare spending in the future because its decisions will automatically take effect unless counteracted by Congress.
As it stands today, private insurance already pays more per patient than
Medicare, and more doctors and providers may be pushed to turn to
that higher-paying source.

The Costs of ACA

The Congressional Budget Office states that the ACA should pay for
itself. Common sense suggests that insuring 30 million people while
guaranteeing new health care benefits will impose a significant financial burden on taxpayers. The money to pay for the ACA will be generated by cutting spending in existing programs such as Medicare and by
creating new taxes, fees, and penalties that individuals, employers, and
the health care industry will have to pay.

One of the biggest sources of revenue for the ACA, besides Medicare
spending cuts, will be an increase in the Medicare hospital insurance
tax that workers pay. The current tax is 2.90 percent, with the employer
and employee each contributing 1.45 percent. The ACA raises the
employee portion to 2.35 percent for high-income earners, specifically
for individuals who make more than $200,000 per year and for couples
who make more than $250,000 per year.

Another source of revenue will come from the Medicare contribution tax imposed on high-income earners. This new 3.8 percent tax will
apply only to investment income, such as capital gains, interest, divi-
dends, annuities, royalties, and rents above the income thresholds.

The pharmaceutical and health insurance industries also face new
fees, which they accepted because of their anticipated profit from the
ACA.

The IRS will enforce a tax penalty of $95 or 1 percent of your income
(whichever is greater) in calendar year 2014 if you do not have health
insurance. The penalty will increase to $695 or 2.5 percent of your
income (whichever is greater) in calendar year 2016. There are exemptions from the individual mandate for certain religious groups, Native
Americans, and people who face a financial hardship that precludes

them from purchasing health insurance. The tax is calculated for each noncovered month at 1/12 of the annual amount in effect.

The ACA imposes a 40 percent tax on expensive health insurance plans, effective in 2018. Health insurance plans that exceed $10,200 in premiums for an individual or $27,500 for a family (excluding dental and vision) will be taxed at a rate of 40 percent above the threshold. These numbers are not very high, and they are not adjusted upward for inflation. As of 2012, employers were required for the first time to list the value of the health insurance they provide on employees' IRS W-2 forms.

The ACA increases the tax penalty from 10 percent to 20 percent for nonallowable purchases made using tax-deductible funds in health savings accounts and flexible spending accounts. As of 2011, health savings accounts and flexible spending accounts may be used only to purchase prescription drugs and can no longer be used for over-the-counter drugs unless you first obtain a prescription from the doctor for the over-the-counter drug. As of 2013, an employer's tax-free contribution to an employee's flexible savings account is limited to $2,500 maximum per year, where it previously was unlimited.

In 2013, the medical deduction threshold was increased from 7.5 percent to 10 percent. This will apply to those age sixty-five and older beginning in 2017.

In conclusion, supporters of the ACA believe it pursues a worthy goal of expanding health care coverage to those who cannot afford it. Detractors are concerned about many factors, including the unintended consequences yet to occur. Regardless of your political views on the new law, one thing is clear: significant health care changes have already been set in motion that will touch just about everyone.

CHAPTER NINE

Plan Your Estate

In dealing with a loved one's incapacity or death, many people discover laws they do not understand or that they never even knew about. Mistakes can be costly, and not putting together a plan can have serious financial consequences. In this chapter, we provide information that we hope will help you understand some of your options so that you can avoid mistakes and take steps that are right for you and your loved ones.

Trusts

Many people do not understand what a trust can accomplish. Trusts are a fundamental planning tool that can give you flexibility to manage your assets before and after death. They can allow you to avoid the cost and delay of probate. But not all trusts are the same. There are many different types of trusts, and each can accomplish different goals. A trust should be constructed to meet your goals.

In general, a trust is an agreement between the trustor, a trustee, and the beneficiaries. A trustor is the person who creates the trust and transfers property to the trust. The trustee is the person who administers the trust according to the terms of the trust. The beneficiary is the person who benefits from, or will benefit from, the trust. There can be more than one trustor, trustee, or beneficiary of a trust. The successor trustee is the one named to administer the trust when the original trustee or co-trustees become incapacitated or die. A revocable trust can be revoked or amended as stated in the trust document. Once a trust is created, the person who created the trust can transfer title of property owned by that person to the name of the trust.

Last Will and Testament

A last will and testament is a legal document that provides for the distribution of some or all of your property after death. It can be changed or revoked at any time if you are still of sound mind. *Sound mind* simply means you understand that you are executing a will, you know the general nature and extent of your property, and you know the people who would normally be expected to share in your estate. You are not required to give your estate to any of them, although a surviving spouse has some rights.

If you die without a valid will or trust and without transferring your property in some other way (such as through "payable on death," beneficiary designations, or joint ownership), state law will determine how your property will be distributed. This is known as dying *intestate*, which means without a will. In a will, you determine who will receive your property after your death.

Any property you have that passes to someone upon your death through joint ownership, a trust, or a beneficiary designation will not be controlled by your will. Property passing under a will goes through probate. Probate is the court-supervised process that determines the validity of your will and oversees the distribution of assets that pass under your will.

Case Study: Second Marriage Situations

Gary's wife died two years ago. He has two adult children. Gary meets Sally, who is divorced and has three adult children. Gary and Sally decide to marry. They combine all their assets and title all the accounts as joint tenants with rights of survivorship. They buy a house together and take title as joint tenants with rights of survivorship.

A few years later, Garry dies. Sally, the surviving joint tenant, owns all the property outright in her name solely. Sally does not do any planning, and when she dies, all her property passes by the laws of intestacy, which means it is divided equally among her three children. Gary's children get nothing.

Gary and Sally had options to ensure that Gary's children would receive an inheritance. They could have set up a revocable trust and had a portion of the assets in trust become irrevocable at the first death. They could have kept the assets separate, and then each of them could have created an estate plan. Many people think that their estates are modest and that they therefore do not need to do any planning. But this can lead to the children of the first spouse to die receiving nothing.

Nevada is a community property state. Property that is community property, without a will, passes entirely to the surviving spouse. Property that is separate property, without a will, passes according to statute. In a community property state, you have testamentary disposition over only one-half of the community property. This means that you can give away only one-half of the community property unless your spouse consents.

Sara was married to Bruce for many years, and Sara had an account with a beneficiary designation naming her daughter from a prior marriage. Sara did not have Bruce sign a consent to the designation. When Sara died, Bruce was starting to become forgetful, and his children were taking control. Bruce's children had Bruce make a claim to one-half of the account, and the claim was successful.

Family Disputes

Unequal or unusual bequests may lead to family disputes. As a practical matter, the making of unusual bequests of substantial assets increases the likelihood of a legal challenge to your will later on. If you want to make an unusual bequest, it is wise to consider getting legal advice.

People are often vulnerable during their final illness. They come to rely on the person who is providing care, whether it is a family member or a professional. Often the caregiver will begin to urge the vulnerable and dying person to make or change estate-planning documents so that the caregiver receives most or all of the estate. For example, Hilda was frail, and after her husband died, she was distraught. Her caregiver had her sign a beneficiary designation form leaving a large account to the caregiver. A Nevada law is designed to make this result more difficult.

The law provides that a transfer is presumed to be void if the following two conditions exist. First, the transfer is effective on or after the transferror's death. This would include transfers that occur by will, trust, deed, payable-on-death designation, or other beneficiary designation. Second, the person who is to receive the assets is one of the following:

- the person who drafted the transfer instrument
- a caregiver of the transferrer (A caregiver is defined as any person who has provided significant assistance or services to or for a person, regardless of whether the person is incompetent, incapacitated, or of limited capacity, and regardless of whether the person is being compensated for the assistance or services provided.)
- a person who arranged for or paid for the drafting of the transfer instrument
- a person who is related to, affiliated with, or subordinate to any person described above (This means a spouse, a relative in the third degree of consanguinity or the spouse of such a relative, a co-owner of a business, an employee of a business, someone with an ownership interest in the business or a supervisory position in the business, or an attorney or employee of an attorney of whom the person was a client.)

The presumption that the transfer is void will not apply in the following circumstances:

- A will is executed and the beneficiary does not receive more than he or she would have received under the laws of intestacy. For example, if a woman has no spouse and two children, under the laws of intestacy, the two children each receive 50 percent of the estate. The will is presumed void if the caregiver child receives more than 50 percent of the estate, or if the child who receives more than 50 percent of the estate arranged for or paid for the drafting.

- The court determines on clear and convincing evidence that the transfer was not the product of fraud, duress, or undue influence.
- The transfer instrument is reviewed by an independent attorney who meets with the person and signs a certificate of independent review stating that the transfer is not a product of fraud, duress, or undue influence.
- The beneficiary is a charitable entity.
- The amount transferred is less than three thousand dollars.

Updating Your Documents

If you already have a will or trust, make sure it still works for you. Wills and trusts do not expire, but your changing family and circumstances may warrant updating your documents. In thinking about your estate plan, it is important to look at all the components of your financial plan and see the big picture.

If you become a resident of a new state, your will or trust should still work, but differences in the law can create problems, so have your documents reviewed by a qualified lawyer. Powers of attorney should also be reviewed. Coordinate who will inherit what, both under your will or trust and outside probate. Make sure your entire estate is distributed as you planned.

Gifts and Loans

Giving your property away before death is another estate-planning option, as are loans that are forgiven upon death. These strategies have significant tax implications and can create serious problems for future eligibility for public benefits, such as Medicaid long-term care benefits. It would be wise to obtain proper legal and tax advice. If you make a gift, be clear about whether it is an advancement on an inheritance. If you make a loan, be clear about the terms for repayment. If the unpaid balance is to be forgiven, is the forgiven amount to be part of that beneficiary's share of the estate? Do not hide what you are doing. Be clear and document it. Ideally, loans should be in writing and signed and notarized.

Special Situations

To ensure your minor children, disabled children, elderly parents, and pets are taken care of in accordance with your wishes, you should plan ahead.

If you leave assets directly to a minor child, then a legal guardian of the child's estate must be appointed to manage the child's affairs. A guardian is someone who has the legal authority and duty to care for another person or property because of minority, incapacity, or disability. You can nominate, or appoint, a guardian for your children, rather than have the court select one for you.

Several things are important to consider when making plans for a guardian. You should consult with the person you name to be sure he or she wants the job, and name an alternative guardian in case your first choice changes his or her mind or dies before the child is grown. Discuss with the guardian your views on education, moral upbringing, religion, and any other matters important to you. In Nevada, you can appoint the guardian in your will or other document, and the court may then formally appoint the named person as guardian at the time needed and upon a proper petition filed with the court.

Trusts, which enable property to be used and managed properly for a beneficiary, can be very helpful in planning for the care of a disabled child or other person with a disability. However, trust planning must be handled carefully in cases where the disabled individual relies on public benefits, such as Medicaid or Supplemental Security Income. An outright distribution of assets to the disabled individual, or general instructions to use the trust for support, could cause the disabled individual to lose eligibility for public benefits. In these situations, a special needs trust should be considered. A special needs trust allows the beneficiary to receive goods or services paid for by the trust, without jeopardizing his or her eligibility for public benefits. The trust supplements public benefits.

The law imposes strict requirements and limitations on these kinds of trusts. Therefore, you should have an attorney experienced not only in trust law, but also in Medicaid, social security, and public benefits law, give you advice and draft the trust. Any trustee appointed should also have some understanding of the relevant public benefits programs.

We often hear, "I love my daughter, but I do not like her husband. How can I help my daughter without him getting his hands on the money?" Or, "My son is just not good with money. What can I do?" To protect beneficiaries from themselves, their creditors, their spouses, and others, consider establishing a spendthrift trust. In such a trust, money is set aside and managed for a particular beneficiary rather than given to them outright. Properly established spendthrift trusts prevent the beneficiary's creditors, spouses, and future lawsuits from reaching the funds. This money will be used for the benefit of the beneficiary in the ways you direct—for example, to pay for education or as a down payment on a home.

The most important thing to consider when establishing a spendthrift trust is who will be the trustee, overseeing the management of the assets. The trustee should be someone you trust, someone familiar with your values and what you would like to see done with the money, and someone who can say "no" to the beneficiary.

Nevada law allows for pet trusts, through which a pet owner can set aside a sum of money to care for a pet if the owner dies or is incapacitated. When creating a pet trust, make sure to include specific instructions for feeding, housing, and veterinary care. Name the individual who will care for your pet as well as an alternate. Specify the amount of money you put in the trust, which should be sufficient to care for the pet as directed.

Another option is to endow a pet with a set sum of money. For instance, many shelters require a life-care endowment to provide for pets until their natural death. A similar gift provision can name a specific person and an alternate to receive a living pet of a deceased person with a set amount of money to cover food and veterinary costs.

Deed upon Death

Under Nevada law, an owner or owners of real property (the grantor or grantors) may execute a deed that conveys their interest in the property to a beneficiary or to multiple beneficiaries upon the owner's death. This deed is usually called a *deed upon death* or *beneficiary deed.* The deed upon death is valid only if executed and recorded in the county where the property is located before the death of the owner or the death of the last surviving owner. A deed upon death may be revoked at any time by the owner, using the appropriate form. If the owner transfers the real property to another person during the owner's lifetime, the deed upon death is void.

If a probate is filed and the owner's probate estate is insufficient to satisfy allowed claims, the property or properties transferred by a deed upon death may be subject to claims against the owner's estate under certain circumstances. The proceeding to enforce the claim must be commenced no later than eighteen months after the owner's death.

A beneficiary inherits the property subject to any liens on the property. When the property is transferred to multiple beneficiaries, the beneficiaries will have to cooperate with each other to sell or manage the property. A deed upon death does not limit Medicaid from recovering benefits paid on behalf of the owner.

Nevada Asset Protection Trust

Many people are looking to protect their hard-earned assets from creditors. Nevada has very favorable laws to protect those who have taken steps before a claim arises. An excellent method of asset protection is to set up a self-settled spendthrift trust, sometimes called a Nevada Asset Protection Trust.

Nevada is one of thirteen states that permit you to create a trust for your benefit that you control and that protects assets from creditors. It takes two years before the asset protection becomes effective, and that is two years from the time assets are transferred to the trust, not two years from the time the trust was created.

The requirements of setting up a Nevada Asset Protection Trust are simple. It must be in writing and be irrevocable. The trustee cannot be required to make any distribution to a beneficiary, meaning that all distributions are purely in the discretion of the trustee. All or part of the assets must be held in Nevada. If you are the trustee and the beneficiary, you or another trustee must be a Nevada resident.

This means that these trusts can be used for people living outside the state of Nevada. Nevada laws can be used to protect assets regardless of the state of residence, provided a friend, relative, bank, or other trusted person resides in Nevada and serves as a trustee. Also, the requirement of having Nevada assets can be met by creating a Nevada family limited partnership or a Nevada limited-liability company that holds the assets.

Assets in a Nevada Asset Protection Trust are still considered available for Medicaid and VA purposes, so while this is a great tool for general asset protection, it cannot be used solely for long-term care purposes. Hybrid strategies can combine the benefits of an asset-protection trust with asset protection from the costs of long-term care.

A 2010 article in *Forbes* magazine gave letter grades to the states that permitted self-settled asset-protection trusts. Nevada led the list as the only state to receive an A+. Among the reasons for the highest grade are that Nevada has no income tax, only a two-year waiting period, and no statutory exceptions for creditors to pierce the trust. When timed well and carefully structured, a Nevada Asset Protection Trust can provide significant creditor protection for one's assets.

Protecting Your Legal Documents

To protect important legal documents and prevent confusion and delay, you should organize these documents, store them in a safe location, and let people know where they are kept.

Some of the important legal documents that should be kept include the following:

- adoption papers
- birth certificate
- citizenship papers, if not born a U.S. citizen
- death certificate of a spouse
- designation of guardian
- divorce papers
- do-not-resuscitate orders
- durable power of attorney for health care
- durable power of attorney for financial matters
- last will and testament
- living will
- marriage certificate
- prenuptial agreements
- trust documents
- veteran's discharge documents

Original legal documents should be stored in a safe place at home or where your family, agent, or legal representative will be able to find them. Some attorneys are willing to store the originals of documents they draft for you, but others will ask you to store the originals.

Copies of your health care advance directives should be given to your health care decision maker, doctor, and other health care providers. In Nevada, they may also be filed with the Secretary of State's Living Will Lockbox. See LivingWillLockbox.com for forms.

Once you have collected and stored all your important legal documents in a safe and accessible location, it is important to let people know where they are. If you have documents stored in a safe deposit box, be sure to include the names of the signers on the box in your document locator list.

Getting your legal affairs in order when faced with a serious illness or injury is important and takes effort, but you are not alone. Bernard and Barbara were happily married for more than twenty-two years when she suffered a stroke. He obtained an equal division of assets for his financial security. He thought all his legal plans were set in stone when he found out that he had inoperable cancer. It hit him that he would most likely not be around to take care of his wife as he had planned. His documents did have successors named, but his imminent death has caused him to rethink what he wants to do to make sure his wife receives the care and attention he would have provided. Wisely, Bernard has now updated all his documents with very detailed provisions about his wife's care.

After Death

One of the most difficult experiences in life is to lose someone you love. You will deal with many emotional issues. At the same time, you may be faced with legal and financial concerns. You may be shocked at all you have to do, especially while grieving, when it is so difficult to summon up the necessary focus and energy. Getting a handle on the legal and financial issues surrounding the death of a loved one can contribute to your emotional healing. The more you understand about these issues, the more you will be enabled to take the steps that are right for you and your family.

Determine How Assets Are Titled

In determining what happens to a specific asset, it is necessary to ascertain how that asset is titled. Generally, only property in the sole name of the decedent at the time of death is subjected to the probate process. Property held in trust or joint tenancy or as community property with the rights of survivorship, accounts bearing "payable on death," "in trust for," or "transfer on death" designations do not require probate. Property passing by contract through the use of a beneficiary designation does not require probate unless the beneficiary named is the estate, is predeceased and there is no contingent beneficiary, or has been disinherited by operation of law. Assets held by contract are those such as life insurance, IRAs, and annuities. Assets held as tenants in common do require a probate because the decedent retains the right to dispose of the interest. Pending lawsuits will also be included in the estate.

Joint Tenancy. Assets held in joint tenancy pass directly to the surviving joint tenant(s) without the need for probate. The surviving joint tenant(s) should take steps to remove the name of the decedent from the asset. For real property, a surviving joint tenant should have an affidavit terminating joint tenancy prepared and recorded. For bank accounts, a surviving joint tenant should present a certified death certificate to the bank and request removal of the deceased joint tenant's name. Alternatively, the account may be closed and all the proceeds withdrawn. For vehicles, a surviving joint tenant should present a certified death certificate at the Department of Motor Vehicles and will need to complete the appropriate forms. For manufactured homes, the surviving joint tenant should present a certified death certificate to the Department of Manufactured Housing.

Payable on Death and Transfer on Death Property. Many types of financial accounts can have a payable on death or transfer on death designation. These accounts will pass directly to the named beneficiary without the need for probate. The named beneficiary should send a death certificate and a letter of instruction directly to the financial institution with instructions on distribution. For real property with a beneficiary deed recorded on the property, one of the named beneficiaries should record an affidavit of death of grantor along with a certified death certificate.

IRAs, Annuities, and Life Insurance. These types of assets frequently have a named beneficiary and will pass directly to the named beneficiary without the need for probate. The named beneficiary should send a certified death certificate and a letter of instruction directly to the financial institution with instructions on distribution. If the named beneficiary is deceased, or there is no named beneficiary, then the asset would be subject to the probate process.

Trust Assets. For assets titled in a trust, the successor trustee will need to administer those assets according to the terms of the trust and according to law.

Community Property. Under Nevada community property laws, each spouse has the power to bequeath only his or her one-half share of the marital property and all his or her separate property. The survivor already owns his or her one-half share, and thus keeps that share. The surviving spouse is the presumptive owner of half of all property acquired during marriage.

The decedent's share, to the extent it has not passed by other methods such as trusts, joint tenancy, or beneficiary designations, will be subject to probate. In Nevada, community property can be held as *community property with right of survivorship.* The effect of this titling is that the asset passes to the surviving spouse.

All income and assets obtained during the marriage are considered community property except those acquired by gift or inheritance. There is a presumption that all property in either spouse's name is community property, although this presumption can be overcome by showing that the property was brought into the marriage or received as a gift or an inheritance. Typically, a written agreement will be used to convert community property to separate property. A prenuptial agreement can also be used to change the community property rules.

Probate Process

For estates not exceeding $20,000, when the property is titled solely in the name of the decedent without any beneficiary designation, and when there is no real property in Nevada, the property may be passed by an affidavit of entitlement. This avoids the need for a probate but does not apply to real estate no matter its value. At least forty days must have passed since the decedent's death.

If the total value of assets held solely in the decedent's name, without a beneficiary designation, exceeds $20,000, a probate is necessary. Assets that do not go through probate include those held in joint tenancy or in a trust, life insurance or retirement accounts with beneficiary designations, and assets with a payable on death designation.

Probate is a legal process for settling the debts of someone who has died, and ensuring the assets go to the proper heirs. During the probate process, the court appoints the person to administer the estate, who then must follow specific statutory obligations. If there is a will, the court will validate the will and settle any disputes or will contests. If there is no will, the statute determines who the heirs are.

If a person dies with assets in his or her name but with no beneficiary named, those assets will go through probate. A will does not avoid probate. If you have a will, probate is the only way to transfer property after death if the asset is only in your name with no named beneficiary.

In probate, a summary administration is for estates not exceeding $200,000, and a full administration is for estates exceeding $200,000. If the net value of the assets (fair market value of probate assets less mortgages and liens but not unsecured debts) is over $20,000 but less than $100,000, a petition to set aside the estate may be filed. If a probate is required, you will need to take the following steps.

— *File the Will.* The original will and codicils, if any, must be filed with the Clerk of the Court within thirty days from the date of death.

—*File the Appropriate Petition.* The appropriate petition must be filed in probate court to appoint the personal representative or, if there is no will, the administrator. The Nevada Revised Statutes state which family members have priority to serve as the administrator when there is no will or trust. The administrator must be a Nevada resident or serve as co-administrator with a Nevada resident. If the value of the gross estate does not exceed $200,000, the court may enter an order granting summary administration. If it is later discovered that the estate exceeded $200,000, the personal representative must petition the court to revoke the summary administration status and order full administration.

—*Obtain Letters Testamentary.* Once appointed as personal representative under a will, you should obtain certified copies of letters testamentary issued by the Clerk of the Court evidencing your authority to act on behalf of the estate. During the course of administration, you will be required from time to time to present copies of the letters to persons with whom you transact estate business. If there is no will, then you obtain letters of administration, which will give you authority to act on behalf of the estate.

— *Follow Your Fiduciary Duty.* As personal representative, you will be required to observe the standards in dealing with the estate assets that would be observed by a prudent person dealing with the property of another. You are under a duty to settle and distribute the estate in an expeditious and efficient manner as is consistent with the best interests of the estate. Any sale or encumbrance of any estate property to yourself, your spouse, your agent, or any corporation, entity, or trust in which you have a substantial beneficial interest is voidable by any person interested in the estate unless the transaction is approved by the court.

— *Prepare and File the Inventory.* Compile an inventory of all assets and obtain valuation of the assets as of the date of death. You will need to file the inventory with the probate court sixty days after the appointment of the personal representative or administrator.

—*Send Notice to Creditors.* Compile a list of all the debts of the decedent. A "Notice to Creditors" should be published in a local newspaper. This will cut off the claims of any creditors who fail to file a claim. To be valid as a charge against the assets of the estate, a creditor's claim must be presented within sixty days (for summary administration) or ninety days (for full administration) after the first publication of the notice. You should not make any distributions of assets until the Notice to Creditors period has expired and all other aspects of estate administration are completed.

— *Open Estate Checking Account.* It is generally best to open an estate checking account and pay all bills from this account so you can track all expenditures. The account needs to be a new account in the name of the estate, not the continuation of an account owned by the decedent. You will need to obtain an EIN number from the IRS before you can open the estate account.

— *File Tax Returns.* You must file the final income tax return for the decedent. If the decedent has a surviving spouse, he or she may file a joint tax return for the previous year. You may also need to file an income tax return for the estate, a trust income tax return, and a federal estate tax return.

— *File Final Account.* You must file a final account with the probate court listing any income to the estate since the date of death, all expenses, and changes in value of assets. The final account can be submitted after the Notice to Creditors period has expired. Once the probate court approves the final account, and after the debts have been paid, any tax returns prepared and any taxes paid, and expenses of administration paid, the personal representative or administrator can distribute the assets to the heirs. Distribution to heirs cannot be made without a court order.

— *Obtain Receipts.* You need to obtain receipts from all heirs who receive any assets. Once you file all the receipts with the probate court, an order of final discharge may be filed with the court.

Avoiding Probate

There are two main reasons to avoid probate: time and expense. An AARP nationwide survey showed that probate typically takes about two years. If your estate is not organized, or if there are family issues, it can take even longer. For those who own property in more than one state, even timeshares, the estate can go through probates in each state involved.

Do not make "My Estate" the beneficiary of retirement plans, an IRA, annuities, or life insurance because this makes the asset subject to probate. If your beneficiary has special needs, you should create a trust and make the trust the beneficiary of those types of assets. Probate can be avoided through the use of a properly funded trust.

Tips for the Surviving Spouse

These steps can help you streamline the estate settlement process and ensure that your spouse's wishes are honored and your needs met.

1. Locate and review your spouse's legal documents, including wills, trusts, and related documents.

2. Identify your spouse's assets and liabilities. Financial assets include checking, savings, and brokerage accounts; pensions; retirement programs; and life insurance. Obligations include mortgages, auto and personal loans, and unpaid credit card balances.

3. Locate and review deeds and titles to real property such as cars and boats.

4. Research and apply for any social security, medical, or other benefits that may be available to you as a surviving spouse. If your spouse was working, contact your spouse's employer to learn about retirement plans (profit sharing, pension, 401[k], 403[b], ESOP) in which your spouse was participating.

5. Meet with the estate's personal representative or attorney, if appropriate, to discuss legal and tax issues associated with settling the estate.

6. Identify and review all insurance policies (e.g., life, home, auto, and personal property) that your spouse owned and notify the respective companies of the death. Contact the insurance companies to ensure that the property will still be covered while you manage your spouse's affairs. Many carry additional benefits in the event of accidental death—some life insurance policies may double the policy coverage amount.

7. Notify your spouse's credit card companies of the death and cancel his or her cards. Be sure to ask whether any death benefits are associated with the card. Many companies provide accidental death insurance, which pays off credit balances in the event of death.

8. Transfer assets to beneficiaries. Contact all the institutions holding the financial assets you have identified. Each will have its own set of requirements on how to transfer assets to beneficiaries. Most will require a death certificate.

Places to Look for Records

- Files. Check the person's physical file and look for any records kept on a computer.
- Mail. Check the mail for sixty to ninety days for anything you may have overlooked. Not all financial service firms send regular statements, so continue checking the mail for the next six to twelve months. If the mail is not coming to your address and you are the personal representative, submit a change of address.
- Tax returns. The deceased's tax returns for the previous two years should identify any assets or tax credits carried over from previous tax periods.
- Safe deposit box. Check any safe deposit boxes for documents.
- Address book. Contact attorneys, accountants, or financial advisors listed in the address book of the deceased.

Moving Forward

This book is intended to help you find ways to make caregiving a positive experience. Whether you are caring for your elders, are a senior citizen yourself, or are preparing for your later years, the goal is to achieve the best health and quality of life possible.

Our aging population is demonstrating a capacity for vigor and independence long after retiring. It is a myth that older persons live out their final years in nursing homes, sick and miserable. The majority of older persons live in the community with strong bonds to their families.

Caregiving can be a stressful time that affects the lives of all concerned, emotionally, financially, and physically. It is an adjustment to accept help and an adjustment to offer help. Choosing to ask for help will allow continued independence, and choosing to accept the role of caregiver and all it implies will be an affirming moment for the family.

How we care for our elders will be with us long after our duties are over. You will always know that you did, perhaps not a perfect job, but the best you could to repay all they have given to you. In the words of

Dr. Robert Niemeyer, "Sometimes the richest things can come into our lives from places that we would never chose to go."

Let the information in this book be an important tool to help you remain in control and avoid living in a world of crisis intervention as your family takes this important journey through the aging process.

Guide to the Family Meeting

Ideally, a family meeting should take place before there is a family crisis. It should include all family members, especially your elder family members. This meeting is all about them, and they should have the major decision-making role if possible. If your loved one has advanced dementia and cannot understand the purpose of the meeting, or if such a family gathering will be upsetting, he or she should not be included. Here are some guidelines for an effective family meeting:

1. Arrange a time that is convenient to most. Use someone's home, if available, or a conference room, if a family member has access to one. The setting should be quiet and as neutral as possible.

2. Everyone who has an interest should be involved. Use a conference call if some members cannot be at the meeting in person and a record the call in case some family members are not available by phone.

3. Develop an agenda before the meeting. A sample agenda is provided below. Send the agenda before the meeting so that all family members can begin to think about the issues and educate themselves about resources they may need to tap. Ask your family if there is something they would like to see as an agenda item. If family members cannot attend, see if you can get their written ideas about agenda items so that those can be read as each topic is discussed.

4. Name a leader or a facilitator to conduct the meeting and

keep it on track. This person must be able to put aside his or her own issues with family members and act evenly and openly with all. Think of the person in your family you would choose if you were all jury members and you needed a foreman.

5. If family dynamics will interfere with the success of the meeting, hire a professional facilitator to take command and keep the meeting from disintegrating into chaos and anger. A qualified family therapist, social worker, mediator, or geriatric care manager will be able to act as a neutral anchor.

6. Have someone keep notes on the meeting so that your decisions on record and can be sent to each participating member.

7. If the family does not have a professional working with them, it may be a good idea to give a specific task to each member. For example, Jane can investigate assisted living facilities, Mary can look into the cost and feasibility of home care, and John can find out what legal issues need to be addressed.

8. Set the boundaries before the meeting. Everyone must be courteous. There will be no accusations of who did what to whom or who was loved the most. Everyone must be allowed to speak without interference. If a family member says he or she cannot participate in some caregiving issue, others cannot respond negatively. There is no use in "demanding" a member take on a responsibility that he or she is not willing to perform. Perhaps the member can think of some other role that will be more acceptable. Family members must agree to listen with an open mind, and all should be willing to meet again, if the agenda is not completed or if more issues crop up as a result of the meeting.

9. If you are a family member with an idea, be ready to back up your notion with facts. For example, if you think your mother needs more care in the home, explain how the additional care will have a positive effect on her life. Make suggestions about how to get the extra care and how much it will cost.

10. If the family cannot agree on all issues, note the ones that have been settled and agree to have another meeting on the issues

still open. Set a time and a place for the next meeting. Reiterate what has been accomplished by this meeting and what remains to be done.

Sample Agenda

Each family's meeting will have a different agenda, depending on the specific issues they face. Here is a sample of a family meeting agenda that you can use as a starting point:

1. Introduction. The facilitator should conduct the meeting and announce who will be keeping notes and that the notes will be sent to each member after the meeting. The facilitator can explain the purpose of the meeting and then ask for comments after each agenda item or give an overview first and then ask for comments. We suggest the latter so that you do not get bogged down on one item and never get to hear the entire plan.

2. Purpose of meeting. State the major concerns that bring the family together. Is it to plan for the future, or is there a crisis at hand that needs immediate attention? What are the goals of the meeting?

3. History. The facilitator should give a brief overview of the elder's present situation. This should include the level of assistance he or she requires at this time and how and if those needs are being met. You can break this down into:

- medical needs and cognitive needs
- physical needs
- safety requirements
- activities of daily living
- instrumental activities of daily living
- legal needs, such as trusts, advanced directives, DNRs, durable power of attorney

4. Discussion. Here are questions to discuss:

- What can family members realistically do to assist with the caregiving needs required?

- What are the pivotal needs that must be accomplished as soon as possible?
- Are there any other concerns that family members think need to be discussed?
- What caregiving resources are being used now, and who will look into what resources are available as needs increase?
- What about alternative living arrangements?
- If your loved one needs more care, the family needs to talk about the possibly of placement in an assisted living setting or a nursing home. Should that be in the area where the elder lives now, or should they move closer to a family member? Which family member? Who would be willing to act as the closest relative? Who has the time, the patience, or the motivation to take on the major caregiving role?

5. Specific tasks assigned to each member.
   - Which family members agree to what specific tasks?
   - Who will be the primary caregiver dealing with hands-on care and who will be the family spokesperson with health care professionals?
   - Who will make sure the legal needs are addressed?
   - Who will take financial responsibility if the elder cannot be responsible?
   - Who will make sure that the elder has the emotional and spiritual support he or she needs?
   - Who will be in charge of dealing with Medicare, Medicaid, or VA benefits to make sure there are no gaps in service and that all resources are being used?

Concluding the Meeting

It may very well be that one member of the family will take on more than one role and that another may not be able to do much at all. There should be no finger pointing or lecturing about this. You can only ask for, not demand, participation. If a daughter is willing only to make one telephone call a week and another can give respite to the primary care-giver every other weekend, so be it.

Make sure the members understand that their roles and tasks are to start immediately and that they can report back to the family on how they are doing and what further needs to be done at the next meeting.

Resource Guide

This guide provides caregivers with useful resources and information, with a focus on Nevada. In this changed economy, despite an increased demand for resources, services have declined as a result of budgetary constraints and cutbacks. There is a higher demand for elder protective services to address neglect and financial exploitation, and with fewer resources, families must be diligent and creative.

Although this guide cannot answer all your questions, it should serve as a directory to find further assistance. The information in this guide was correct at the time of publication, but we cannot assume responsibility for changes that occurred thereafter. Additional and updated resource information for Nevada caregivers can be found at www.nevadaadrc.com.

Advocacy and Legal Assistance

City of Sparks Police Department
1701 East Prater Way
Sparks, NV 89434
(775) 353-2231
www.cityofsparks.us
Offers a senior phone patrol that places daily calls to check on the welfare of senior citizens who live alone.

Clark County Family Law Self-Help Center

601 North Pecos Road—First Floor of Family Courts Center

Las Vegas, NV 89101

(702) 455-1500

Provides information and packets to help navigate the legal maze.

Clark County Senior Advocate Program

3900 Cambridge Street, Suite 200

Las Vegas, NV 89119

(702) 455-7051

Provides a central point of contact for referrals, outreach, partnership, and advocacy for senior citizens, senior services, and programs in Clark County.

Clark County Social Service—Neighborhood Justice Center

330 South Third Street, Suite 600

Las Vegas, NV 89101

(702) 455-3898

Helps Clark County residents resolve conflicts at no cost through mediation services and a comprehensive information and referral program.

Elko County Courthouse Self-Help Center

571 Idaho Street

Elko, NV 89801

www.elkonv.com/~fourjdcl

(775) 753-4600

Provides various form packets, which are available online, in person, or by mail.

Guardian Program—Douglas County

(775) 782-9858

Provides a computerized telephone system designed to stay in touch daily with the elderly.

Legal Aid Center of Southern Nevada
725 E. Charleston Blvd.
Las Vegas, NV 89104
(702) 386-1070
Toll Free: (800) 522-1070
  Provides free legal services for low-income residents of Clark
County, Nevada.

Metro Abuse and Neglect
4750 West Oakey Boulevard
Las Vegas, NV 89102
(702) 828-3364
  Investigates claims of abuse, neglect, and exploitation of the elderly.

Nevada Aging and Disability Services Division
3416 Goni Road, Suite D-132
Carson City, NV 89706
(775) 687-4210
www.nvaging.net

  1010 Ruby Vista, Suite 104
  Elko, NV 89801
  (775) 738-1966

  1860 East Sahara Avenue (Regional Office)
  Las Vegas, NV 89104
  (702) 486-3545

  445 Apple Street, Suite 104
  Reno, NV 89502
  (775) 688-2964
  Provides various programs and services, including the following:
  Advocate for Elders—provides advocacy and assistance to frail
seniors, primarily homebound and living in the community; educates
seniors and family members about their rights; and provides informa-

tion and referral regarding programs and services available to home-bound seniors.

Elder Protective Services—receives and investigates complaints of elder abuse.

Long-Term Care Ombudsman Program—protects the rights of the elderly residing in long-term care facilities, including residential group homes.

Nevada Disability Advocacy and Law Center (NDALC)
www.ndalc.org

Elko Office
905 Railroad Street, Suite 104B
Elko, NV 89801
(775) 777-1590

Northern Office
1865 Plumas Street, #2
Reno, NV 89509
(775) 333-7878

Southern Office
6039 Eldora Avenue, Suite C, Box 3
Las Vegas, NV 89146
(702) 257-8150

Offers advocacy services and referral services for individuals with disabilities in Nevada.

Nevada Legal Services
www.nlslaw.net
2621 Northgate Lane, Suite 10
Carson City, NV 89706
(775) 284-3491

380 Court Street, Suite D
Elko, NV 89801
(775) 753-5880

530 South Sixth Street

Las Vegas, NV 89101

(702) 386-0404

204 Marsh Avenue, Suite 101

Reno, NV 89509

(775) 284-3491

Offers free legal services.

Nevada Rural Counties Retired and Senior Volunteer CARE Program

Churchill County (Fallon Lifeline): (775) 423-9406

Elko County (Elko): (775) 753-4060

Humboldt County (Winnemucca): (775) 304-0757

Lincoln County (Caliente): (775) 726-3126

Lyon County (Dayton/Stagecoach): (775) 443-5248

Lyon County (Yerington): (775) 443-5248

Lyon County (Fernley): (775) 575-0717

Lyon County (Dayton/Silver Springs): (775) 443-5248

Mineral County (Schurz): (775) 741-0309

Mineral County (Hawthorne): (775) 945-5911

Nye County (Pahrump): (775) 751-5282

Nye County (Tonopah): (775) 482-6690

Nye County (Gabbs): (775) 772-0332

Esmeralda County (Dyer): (775) 209-2206

Washoe County (Lifeline Program): (775) 787-8186

Storey County (Sparks River District): (775) 342-0264

Storey County (Virginia City): (775) 443-5248

White Pine County (Ely): (775) 289-6323

www.nevadaruralrsvp.org

Provides legal assistance to seniors with end-of-life planning, trusts, living wills, powers of attorney, and various other legal questions. The pro bono attorneys travel the fifteen rural counties of Nevada, volunteering legal services to low-income seniors who are otherwise unable to access such services.

Office of the Governor—Consumer Health Assistance

1100 East William Street, Suite 222
Carson City, NV 89701
(775) 684-3676

555 East Washington Avenue, Suite 4800
Las Vegas, NV 89101
(702) 486-3587
Toll Free: (888) 333-1597

Provides a single point of contact for consumers and injured workers to assist them in disputing medical bills. Provides assistance through information, counseling, education, and advocacy.

Office of the Nevada Attorney General—Medicaid Fraud Control Unit

555 East Washington Avenue, Suite 3900
Las Vegas, NV 89101
(702) 486-3420

100 North Carson Street
Carson City, NV 89701
(775) 684-1191

Investigates Medicaid and Worker's Compensation fraud. Also protects those in long-term care facilities from physical and fiscal abuse and offers legal services.

Senior Citizens Law Program

310 South Ninth Street
Las Vegas, NV 89101
(702) 229-6596

Provides free legal counsel and assistance to Clark County residents age sixty or older on certain matters. Assists with simple wills, advance directives, intervention in elder abuse matters, and powers of attorney. Assists with foreclosures regardless of age.

Senior Legal Hotline

(702) 386-0404

Toll Free: (877) 693-2163

Provides hotline service to assist Nevada residents age sixty years or older.

Volunteer Attorneys for Rural Nevadans

904 North Nevada Street

Carson City, NV 89703

(775) 883-8278

www.varn.org

Provides pro bono representation to individuals of limited means in rural counties.

Washoe County District Court—Family Division

Self-Help Center

1 South Sierra Street

Reno, NV 89501

(775) 325-6731

www.washoecourts.com

Provides form packets, workshops, and information services on family law topics.

Washoe County Senior Citizens Law Center

1155 East Ninth Street

Reno, NV 89512

(775) 328-2592

Provides free legal counsel and assistance to low-income and frail seniors on certain matters.

Washoe Legal Services
299 South Arlington Avenue
Reno, NV 89501
(775) 329-2727
www.washoelegalservices.org
 Provides pro bono representation to Washoe County residents.

Programs and Services

Agai-Dicutta Senior Center
P.O. Box 220
Schurz, NV 89427
(775) 773-2224
 Provides seniors with transportation for shopping and recreation.

Aging and Disability Services
Carson City: (775) 687-4210
Elko: (775) 738-1966
Las Vegas: (702) 486-3545
Reno: (775) 688-2944
www.aging.state.nv.us
 Develops, coordinates, and delivers a comprehensive support service system in order for Nevada's senior citizens to lead independent, meaningful, and dignified lives. It assists seniors in every step of the service continuum from safeguarding their rights, fostering their self-sufficiency, and providing counseling to advocating on their behalf.

Aging and Disability Services—Home and Community–Based Waiver
Carson City: (775) 687-4210
Elko: (775) 738-1966
Las Vegas: (702) 486-3545
Reno: (775) 688-2944
www.nvaging.net

Provides nonmedical services to older individuals to help them maintain independence in their own homes as an alternative to nursing home placement.

Aging and Disability Services—Senior Ride Program
(702) 486-3581

Provides discounted taxicab fares to seniors and persons with disabilities residing in Clark County through coupon booklets that are accepted by all county taxicab companies.

Aging and Disability Services—Waiver for the Elderly in Adult Residential Care (WEARC)

Administration
3416 Goni Road, Suite D-132
Carson City, NV 89706
(775) 687-4210

Elko Regional Office
1010 Ruby Vista Drive, Suite 104
Elko, NV 89801
(775) 738-1966

Las Vegas Regional Office
1860 East Sahara Avenue
Las Vegas, NV 89104
(702) 486-3545

Reno Regional Office
445 Apple Street, Suite 104
Reno, NV 89502
(775) 688-2964

Provides nonmedical, personal care service in a group care setting as a less-expensive alternative.

Battle Mountain Band Council

37 Mountain View Drive

Battle Mountain, NV 89820

(775) 635-2004

Provides seniors with transportation for medical appointments.

Cambridge Community Center

3930 Cambridge Street

Las Vegas, NV 89119

(702) 455-7169

Acts as a central hub for community resources and services.

Care Chest of Sierra Nevada

7910 North Virginia Street

Reno, NV 89506

(775) 829-2273

www.carechest.com

Provides free medical equipment and emergency prescriptions for low-income residents of Nevada.

Catholic Charities of Southern Nevada

Senior Core Program, Respite Service, Retired and Senior Volunteer Program, Senior Companion Program, Telephone Reassurance Program

531 North 30th Street, Suite C

Las Vegas, NV 89101

(702) 382-0721

Provides a cost-effective service that promotes self-sufficiency for elderly clients while providing support and relief for their families. Provides meaningful volunteer opportunities to older persons with limited income. Offers scheduled, regular telephone contact, providing a type of lifeline for individuals living alone. Provides companionship, light housekeeping, light meal preparation, medication reminders, overnight stays, home condition monitoring, help with errands, and incidental transportation. Available part time at reduced rates.

Catholic Charities of Southern Nevada—Meals on Wheels (MOWs)

531 North Thirtieth Street
Las Vegas, NV 89101
(702) 385-5284

Provides meals to qualified seniors who are sixty or older and homebound.

Center for Cognitive Aging

University of Nevada School of Medicine
890 Mill Street, Suite 102
Reno, NV 89502
(775) 322-2731

Provides diagnosis, treatment, counseling, education, and social services to families of people with memory impairments.

CenturyLink Lifeline Services

330 South Valley View
Las Vegas, NV 89107
(702) 244-7580
www.centurylink.com

Provides discounts to the monthly charge for basic local residential phone service to qualifying low-income subscribers.

Churchill County Senior Center

310 East Court Street
Fallon, NV 89406
(775) 423-7096

Provides home energy assistance programs, emergency assistance for fuel bills, and a Meals on Wheels program free for anyone over sixty.

Clark County Assessor

500 South Grand Central Parkway

Las Vegas, NV 89106

(702) 455-3882

Administers the property-tax exemptions and Senior Citizens Tax Assistance/Rent Rebate Program to individuals meeting certain requirements.

Clark County Homemakers Program

3900 Cambridge Street, Suite 208

Las Vegas, NV 89119

(702) 455-8645

Provides case management and a homemaker to income-qualified individuals. Individuals are not required to need personal help. The waiting list for the program without personal help may be longer.

Clark County Housing Authority—Senior Services Program

5390 East Flamingo Road

Las Vegas, NV 89122

(702) 451-8041, ext. 1660

www.haccnv.org/index.htm

Provides information, referral, and assistance to senior and disabled residents living in Clark County Housing Authority (HUD) properties.

Clark County Social Service—Alternative Health Care Program

3900 Cambridge Street, Suite 108

Las Vegas, NV 89119

(702) 455-8646

Promotes the resumption of independent living by providing temporary home health aides to assist recuperating individuals discharged from hospitals and nursing homes.

Clark County Social Service—Community Resource Center
2432 North Martin Luther King, Building D
North Las Vegas, NV 89032
(702) 455-4270

Provides eligibility determination for medical assistance, as well as information about and referrals to other available community services. Social service workers visit Laughlin, Mesquite, Overton, Searchlight, the MASH Crisis Center, and various shelters on request, to determine program eligibility.

Clark County Social Service—Long-Term Care Unit
3900 Cambridge Street
Las Vegas, NV 89119
(702) 455-8687

Provides long-term care placement services to assist in securing appropriate long-term care for Clark County residents who are unable to function in independent living.

Clark County Social Service—Medical Assistance
1600 Pinto Lane
Las Vegas, NV 89106
(702) 455-4270

Provides care to low-income individuals not eligible for other public or private programs. Client services include outpatient clinic care, inpatient hospital care, institutional care, adult day care, medical transportation, and pharmacy services.

Clark County Social Service—Medical Outreach
1600 Pinto Lane
Las Vegas, NV 89106
(702) 455-3052

Assists with discharge planning for patients at University Medical Center of Southern Nevada and local private hospitals and assesses patient eligibility for agency programs at various locations. Staff also visits homebound clients to assess eligibility for agency programs.

Clark County Social Service—Volunteer Program

1600 Pinto Lane
Las Vegas, NV 89106
(702) 455-5719

Recruits and places volunteers in various agency activities, including mentoring teenagers and adults, conducting mediations, providing companionship, performing home maintenance and repairs for seniors, translating, greeting clients, and providing clerical assistance.

Cleveland Clinic Lou Ruvo Center for Brain Health

888 West Bonneville Avenue
Las Vegas, NV 89106
(702) 483-6000

Advances research and treatment of neurodegenerative diseases such as Alzheimer's, Parkinson's, Huntington's, and amyotrophic lateral sclerosis.

The Continuum Outreach Program

Nevada Care Connection Partner
3700 Grant Drive, #A
Reno, NV 89509
(775) 829-4700
http://continuumreno.com

Provides adult day care, therapy, and rehabilitation services.

Daybreak Program

1155 East Ninth Street
Reno, NV 89512
(775) 328-2591
www.washoecounty.us/seniorsrv/daycare.htm

Provides adult day care for the elderly or disabled, including recreation, meals, and therapy.

Dayton Senior Center
320 Old Dayton Valley Road
Dayton, NV 89403
(775) 246-6210
   Provides home energy assistance programs, emergency assistance for fuel bills for seniors, and daily lunches on a donation basis.

Douglas County Senior Services
2300 Meadow Lane
Gardnerville, NV 89410
   Mailing Address:
   P.O. Box 218
   Minden, NV 89423
   (775) 783-6455
www.douglascountynv.gov
   Provides leadership, needs assessment, information exchange, networking, and service advocacy.

East Valley Family Services
1800 East Sahara Avenue
Las Vegas, NV 89104
(702) 631-7098
www.eastvalleyfamilyservices.org
   Helps families and seniors gain and maintain self-sufficiency.

Emergency Aid for Boulder City
600 Nevada Highway
Boulder City, NV 89005
(702) 293-0332
   Provides emergency aid for transients and for utilities, medical care, and automobile gasoline for Boulder City residents only.

Food Bank of Northern Nevada
550 Italy Drive
McCarran, NV 89434

(775) 331-3663

www.fbnn.org

Distributes food to local pantries so that individuals can receive a bag of groceries and other emergency food assistance.

Give me A Break, Inc.

P.O. Box 620721

Las Vegas, NV 89162

(702) 898-2219

www.givemeabreakinc.com

Volunteer respite services including transportation, companionship, and help with shopping.

Helping Hands of Henderson

1125 American Pacific Drive, Suite G

Henderson, NV 89015

(702) 616-6554

Assists the frail, elderly, and disabled with nonmedical needs, such as transportation, wheelchair access, interpreter service, and minor home repairs.

Helping Hands of Vegas Valley, Inc.

2320 Paseo Del Prado, Suite B112

Las Vegas, NV 89102

(702) 633-7264

Provides volunteer-escorted transportation for frail seniors age sixty or older to medical appointments, shopping, and errands in order for them to remain independent as long as possible. The Senior Ride Program provides discounted taxicab coupons that are accepted by many taxi companies in Las Vegas, Henderson, and Pahrump.

HELP of Southern Nevada

1640 East Flamingo Road, #100

Las Vegas, NV 89119

(702) 369-4357

www.helpsonv.org

Provides various services to the community and seniors, such as the no-cost weatherization program.

Hope Link

178 Westminster Way

Henderson, NV 89015

(702) 566-0576

Provides a Senior Community Program called THERE, The Homebound Elderly Recreation Experience. A community advocate will come to the applicant's home and do a needs assessment. If the senior is accepted, a volunteer will come out twice a month and work with him or her on reading, crafts, watching movies, or other interests.

James Seastrand Helping Hands of North Las Vegas, Inc.

3640 North 5th Street, Suite 130

North Las Vegas, NV 89032

(702) 649-7853

Provides escorted transportation for frail elderly and handicapped persons. Also offers respite care, telephone reassurance, referral service, and transportation.

Jewish Family Service Agency

4794 South Eastern Avenue, Suite C

Las Vegas, NV 89119

(702) 732-0304

Provides social service and counseling to all of Clark County, offering referral and case management services, burial and bereavement services, volunteer opportunities, limited financial assistance, and some emergency food assistance.

Lend-a-Hand, Inc.
400 Utah Street
Boulder City, NV 89005
(702) 294-2363

Provides assistance for frail, elderly, or chronically ill and disabled persons of Boulder City so that they may remain in their own homes as long as possible. Services include transportation; respite care; and referral service for light housekeeping, simple home repairs and upkeep, pet walking, meal preparation, and bill assistance. Sliding-scale donation applies.

Lend-a-Hand Senior Services
145 Mount Rose Street
Reno, NV 89509
(775) 322-8414

Offers respite nonmedical caregiving services, meal preparation, and transportation to doctors' appointments.

Lincoln County Human Services
P.O. Box 508
Panaca, NV 89042
(775) 728-4477

Provides nutritious meals to the homebound and to seniors at senior centers. Transportation also provided from Lincoln County to Las Vegas, Cedar City, and St. George, Utah.

Lutheran Social Services of Nevada
73 Spectrum Boulevard
Las Vegas, NV 89101
    Mail:
    P.O. Box 2079
    Las Vegas, NV 89125
(702) 639-1730

Provides utility assistance to seniors over the age of sixty-two, food pantry, and assistance with state ID and birth certificate. Must come in to the office for assistance.

Manufactured Housing Division—Lot Rent Subsidy
2501 East Sahara Avenue, Suite 204
Las Vegas, NV 89104
(702) 486-4135

Provides financial aid to qualifying low-income mobile home park residents by paying 25 percent of their monthly space rent.

Neighborhood Housing Services of Southern Nevada
1849 Civic Center Drive
North Las Vegas, NV 89030
(702) 649-0998
www.nwsn.org

Provides assistance to low-income families in locating subsidized apartments, down payment assistance for low-income first-time homeowners, and foreclosure counseling.

Nevada Department of Health and Human Services—Division of Public and Behavioral Health
4150 Technology Way
Carson City, NV 89706
(775) 684-4200
www.health.nv.gov

Protects, promotes, and improves the physical and behavioral health of the people in Nevada.

Nevada Department of Health and Human Services
Nevada Division of Public and Behavioral Health—Community Health Nursing
(775) 684-4006
www.health.nv.gov/CommunityHealthNursing.htm

Each clinic offers a variety of services to residents in Nevada's rural counties.

Nevada Department of Health and Human Services—Division of Welfare and Supportive Services

1470 East College Parkway

Carson City, NV 89706

(775) 684-0500

https://dwss.nv.gov

Administers the Medicaid program for seniors. A list of offices is located in the government office section below.

Nevada Disability Rx Program

Nevada Department of Health and Human Services

3416 Goni Road, Suite B-113

Carson City, NV 89706

(775) 687-4210

Toll Free: (866) 303-6323

http://dhhs.nv.gov/SeniorRx.htm

Helps low-income seniors buy their medications.

Nevada Health Centers

   Amargosa Valley Medical Center

   845 Farm Road

   Amargosa Valley, NV 89020

   (775) 372-5432

   Austin Medical Center

   121 Main Street

   Austin, NV 89310

   (775) 964-2222

   Beatty Medical Center

   250 South Irving Street

   Beatty, NV 89003

   (775) 553-2208

Cambridge Family Health Center

3900 South Cambridge Street

Las Vegas, NV 89119

(702) 307-5415

Carlin Community Health Center

310 Memory Lane

Carlin, NV 89822

(775) 754-2666

Crescent Valley Medical Center

5043 Tenabo Avenue

Crescent Valley, NV 89821

Eastern Family Medical and Dental Center

2212 South Eastern Avenue

Las Vegas, NV 89104

(702) 735-9334

Elko Family Medical and Dental Center

762 14th Street

Elko, NV 89801

(775) 738-5850

Eureka Medical Center

250 South Main Street

Eureka, NV 89316

(775) 237-5313

Jackpot Community Health Center

135 Keno Street

Jackpot, NV 89825

(775) 755-2500

Las Vegas Outreach Clinic

47 West Owens Avenue

North Las Vegas, NV 89030

(702) 307-4635

Martin Luther King Family Health Center

1799 Mount Mariah Drive

Las Vegas, NV 89106

(702) 383-1961

North Las Vegas Family Health Center

2225 Civic Center Drive, Suite 224

North Las Vegas, NV 89030

(702) 214-5948

Sierra Nevada Health Center

3325 Research Way

Carson City, NV 87906

(775) 887-5140

Wendover Community Health Center

925 Wells Avenue

West Wendover, NV 89833

(775) 664-2220

(800) 787-2568

http:/nevadahealthcenters.org

Provides for primary and preventive health care services, through a federal grant program.

Nevada Urban Indians, Inc.

www.nevadaurbanindians.org

Carson City Office

232 East Winnie Lane

Carson, NV 89706

(775) 883-4439

Reno Office

1475 Terminal Way, Suite B

Reno, NV 89502

(775) 788-7600

Provides home health care, elder visits, light housekeeping for elders, drug and alcohol counseling, an emergency food bank, and a health clinic.

Public Administrators and Public Guardians

Carson City
885 East Musser Street, Suite 1028
Carson City, NV 89701
(775) 887-2260

Churchill County
P.O. Box 789
Fallon, NV 89407
(775) 423-5035

Clark County
515 Shadow Lane
Las Vegas, NV 89106
(702) 455-4332

Douglas County
P.O. Box 1059
Minden, NV 89423
(775) 782-6216

Elko County
P.O. Box 25
Elko, NV 89803
(775) 738-3171

Esmerelda County
P.O. Box 339
Goldfield, NV 89013
(775) 485-6352

Eureka County

P.O. Box 556

Eureka, NV 89136

(775) 237-5263

Humboldt County

501 South Bridge Street

Winnemucca, NV 89446

(775) 623-6370

Lander County

P.O. Box 187

Battle Mountain, NV 89820

(775) 635-5195

Lincoln County

P.O. Box 60

Pioche, NV 89043

(775) 962-5171

Lyon County

P.O. Box 745

Yerington, NV 89447

(775) 722-1664

Mineral County

P.O. Box 456

Hawthorne, NV 89414

(775) 312-0512

Nye County

250 Highway 160, Suite 7

Pahrump, NV 89060

(775) 751-4259

Pershing County

P.O. Box 1167

Lovelock, NV 89419

(775) 273-7453

Storey County

P.O. Box 496

Virginia City, NV 89440

(775) 847-0964

Washoe County

P.O. Box 7360

Reno, NV 89510

(775) 861-4000

White Pine County

801 Clark Street, Suite 3

Ely, NV 89301

(775) 293-6565

Public administrators oversee the administration of the estates of deceased persons who have no qualified person willing and able to do so. Public guardians serve individuals who need assistance and have no qualified person to take care of them or their property. They may also oversee the Representative Payee Program.

Rebuilding Together Southern Nevada

611 South 9th Street

Las Vegas, NV 89101

(702) 259-4900

www.rebuildingtogether.org

Rehabilitates the homes of low-income seniors, disabled, and families with young children; includes assistance with plumbing, heating, electric, ramps, grab bar repair, and leaking roofs. Clients must meet HUD income guidelines.

Regional Transportation Commission

600 South Grand Central Parkway, Suite 350

Las Vegas, NV 89106

(702) 676-1500

P.O. Box 30002

Reno, NV 89520

(775) 348-0400

Provides wheelchair-access transportation for medical appointments and shopping.

Regional Transportation Commission Access

600 Sutro Street

Reno, NV 89512

For reservations: (775) 348-5438

Eligibility certification: (775) 348-0477

Provides transportation service for people with disabilities who meet the eligibility criteria.

Renown Health Senior Options

850 Mills Street, Suite 100

Reno, NV 89502

(775) 982-5400

Offers social events, classes on health-related topics, monthly health screenings, a mall-walking program, a senior conversation group, support groups, exercise programs for people with health concerns, and a free blood pressure check.

Salvation Army

Administration Office

2900 Palomino Lane

Las Vegas, NV 89107

(702) 870-4430

Family Services
1581 North Main Street
Las Vegas, NV 89101
(702) 649-8240

Lied Vocational Training
35 West Owens
Las Vegas, NV 89030
(702) 399-4403
Offers financial assistance, emergency food, substance abuse rehabilitation, and volunteer opportunities.

Sanford Center for Aging
University of Nevada, Reno
MS 146
Reno, NV 89557
(775) 784-4774
Offers a variety of programs and services, including RSVP for
Washoe County; UNR interdisciplinary gerontology curriculum; well-
ness program; medication therapy management; Nevada Care Connec-
tion; and Taking Charge.

Senior Citizens of Searchlight, Inc.
575 South Highway 95
Searchlight, NV 89046
(702) 297-1614
Provides nutritious meals to seniors age sixty or older, wheelchair-access transportation, and friendly visitation.

Senior Mental Health Outreach
6161 West Charleston Boulevard
Las Vegas, NV 89146
(702) 486-5730
Provides specialized community outreach programs, including
evaluation, counseling, case management, and referral services. Qual-

ity mental health care may be provided in the home to improve access. Also facilitates the Children of Older Parents Support Group.

Seniors Helping Seniors, Energy Conservation Program

450 East Bonanza Road
Las Vegas, NV 89101
(702) 382-4412

Assists with weatherization of homes for individuals who are age fifty-five or over, or disabled, and meet other eligibility requirements. Closed during the summer.

Silver State Health Insurance Exchange

2310 S. Carson Street
Suite 2
Carson City, NV 89701
(775) 687-9939
http://exchange.nv.gov

Nevada's exchange as created under the Affordable Care Act is designed to increase the number of insured Nevadans by facilitating the purchase and sale of health insurance. The web page to purchase insurance is www.nevadahealthlink.com.

Southern Nevada Adult Mental Health Services

6161 West Charleston
Las Vegas, NV 89146
(702) 486-6000

Provides group and individual counseling services, medical care, psychiatric emergency services, an observation unit, and an inpatient hospital.

Southern Nevada Centers for Independent Living (SNCIL)

www.sncil.org

4100 North Martin Luther King Boulevard, Suite 100
North Las Vegas, NV 89032

(702) 649-3822
2950 South Rainbow Boulevard, Suite 220
Las Vegas, NV 89146
(702) 889-4216

Offers benefits counseling, peer counseling, emergency food and housing assistance by referral, transportation, general information, and referral and advocacy.

Southern Nevada Transit Coalition (Silver Riders)
260 E. Laughlin Civic Drive
Laughlin, NV 89029
(702) 298-4435

Provides seniors with transportation for medical appointments, shopping, or recreation for a nominal fee.

State Health Insurance Program (SHIP)
(702) 486-3478
Toll Free: (800) 307-4444
Salud en Acción
(702) 759-0874 (Spanish)

Supplies free information, counseling, and assistance to Medicare beneficiaries. Informs seniors and Medicare beneficiaries of their rights under Medicare. Reviews present coverage to prevent seniors from paying for unnecessary or duplicate coverage, assists beneficiaries in understanding their health insurance needs and in processing Medicare claims, and makes referrals to various agencies when appropriate. This program is free of charge.

State of Nevada—Client Assistance Program (CAP)
6039 Eldora Avenue, Suite C
Las Vegas, NV 89146
(702) 257-8150

Assists individuals with disabilities who are having trouble with vocational rehabilitation or independent living services. Uses informal means to the extent possible and then can represent the client in administrative or legal hearings.

State of Nevada—Energy Assistance Program
(702) 486-1404

Toll Free: (800) 992-0900

Assists low-income households with their energy costs. Income information is required, and it may take up to forty-five days for eligibility determination. Call for an application, or go to the local electric company for an application, and fill it out and mail as soon as possible.

United Way of Southern Nevada—Volunteer Centers
5830 West Flamingo Road

Las Vegas, NV 89103

(702) 892-2300

www.volunteercentersn.org

Provides resources to individuals and groups to deliver creative solutions to community problems.

Washoe Senior Ride
Regional Transportation Commission

1155 East Ninth Street

Reno, NV 89512

(775) 328-2575

Provides discount vouchers for partial payment of taxi fares and tips.

Associations and Support Groups

AARP Driver Safety Program
Toll Free: (888) 687-2277

www.aarp.org

Provides safe driving instructions to seniors. Call for locations of classes.

AARP Foundation

Senior Community Service Employment Program (SCSEP)

www.aarpmmp.org/worksearch

5450 West Sahara Avenue, Suite 340

Las Vegas, NV 89146

(702) 648-3356

Reno Office

1135 Terminal Way, #102

Reno, NV 89502

(775) 323-2243

Offers a senior employment program for individuals fifty-five and older who have varied experiences and licenses. Examples of work assignments include library services, community beautification, and personal assistance.

Alzheimer's Association

www.alz.org.dsw

www.alz.org.norcal

5190 South Valley View Boulevard, Suite 104

Las Vegas, NV 89118

(702) 248-2770

Toll Free: (800) 272-3900

Reno Office

1301 Cordone Avenue, Suite 180

Reno, NV, 89502

(775) 786-8061

Provides leadership to eliminate Alzheimer's disease through advancements in research while enhancing care and support services for individuals and their families.

American Cancer Society

www.cancer.org

6165 South Rainbow Boulevard

Las Vegas, NV 89119

(702) 798-6877

691 Sierra Rose Drive, Suite A

Reno, NV 89511

(775) 329-0609

Dedicated to eliminating cancer, saving lives, and diminishing suffering from cancer through research, education, advocacy, and service.

American Diabetes Association

5463 South Durango Drive, Suite 100-A

Las Vegas, NV 89113

(702) 369-9995

Toll Free: (800) 342-2383

www.diabetes.org

Dedicated to curing diabetes and to improving the lives of all people affected by diabetes.

American Heart Association

www.americanheart.org

4445 South Jones Boulevard, Suite 1

Las Vegas, NV 89103

(702) 367-1366

1281 Terminal Way

Reno, NV 89502

(775) 332-7065

Toll Free: (800) 242-8721

Provides fund-raising for research (heart disease and stroke) and community education and awareness.

American Lung Association
www.lungusa.org
   3552 West Cheyenne Avenue, #130
   North Las Vegas, NV 89032
   (702) 948-4155

   10615 Double R Boulevard
   Reno, NV 89521
   (775) 829-5864
   Dedicated to preventing lung disease and promoting lung health.

American Parkinson's Disease Association
P.O. Box 81884
Las Vegas, NV 89180
Information and referral: (702) 464-3132
www.apdaparkinsonslasvegas.org
   Offers counseling services, support group meetings, education, health-related fairs and seminars, a referral service, a Spanish interpreter service, and loans of durable medical equipment.

American Red Cross
www.redcross.org
   1771 East Flamingo Road, Suite 206B
   Las Vegas, NV 89119
   (702) 791-3311

   1190 Corporate Boulevard
   Reno, NV 89506
   (775) 856-1000
   Dedicated to helping people prevent, prepare for, and cope with emergencies in their homes, workplace, and communities.

Arthritis Foundation
1368 Paseo Verde Parkway
Henderson, NV 89012

(702) 367-1626

www.arthritis.com

Dedicated to improving lives through leadership in the prevention, control, and cure of arthritis and related diseases.

Bereavement Support Group

Nathan Adelson Hospice

4141 South Swenson Street

Las Vegas, NV 89119

(702) 733-0320

www.nah.org

Provides support services to assist families in the grieving process.

Blind and Visually Impaired Services

1325 Corporate Boulevard

Reno, NV 89502

(775) 823-8140

Blind Center of Nevada

1001 North Bruce Street

Las Vegas, NV 89101

(702) 642-6000

www.blindcenter.org

Provides information, referral, and advocacy for blind and visually impaired adults.

Blindconnect

6375 West Charleston Boulevard, WCL #200

Las Vegas, NV 89146

(702) 631-9009

www.blindconnect.org

Provides information, referral, and peer support for blind and visually impaired adults.

Bureau of Services to the Blind and Visually Impaired
Las Vegas JobConnect
3016 West Charleston Boulevard, Suite 200
Las Vegas, NV 89102
(702) 486-5333
Toll Free: (800) 662-3366
Provides services to the blind, including vocational rehabilitation.

Deaf and Hard of Hearing Advocacy Resource Center
www.dhharc.org
2575 Westwind Road, Suite C
Las Vegas, NV 89102
(702) 363-3323

1150 Corporate Boulevard, Suite 1
Reno, NV 89502
(775) 355-8994
Provides direct consumer assistance and advocacy.

Divorced and Widowed Adjustment, Inc.
P.O. Box 12042
Las Vegas, NV 89112
(702) 735-5544
www.info4nv.org
Provides emotional support to men and women experiencing difficulties brought about by separation, divorce, or death of a loved one. Separate support groups for widowed, separated, and divorced men and women.

Down Syndrome Organization of Southern Nevada
5300 Vegas Drive
Las Vegas, NV 89108
(702) 648-1990
www.dsosn.org
Promotes a positive understanding of Down syndrome in the community.

Isight, Inc.—Center for the Blind

1001 North Bruce Street
North Las Vegas, NV 89030
(702) 642-6000

Provides a place for socializing, friendly companionship and visitation, telephone reassurance, minor home repairs, loan of durable medical equipment, and electronic recycling.

National Multiple Sclerosis Society

5463 South Durango Drive, Suite 115
Las Vegas, NV 89113
(702) 736-7272

4600 Kietzke Lane, #K223
Reno, NV 89502
(775) 329-7180

Serves those with multiple sclerosis, offering legal service, peer counseling service, loan of durable medical equipment, and a referral service.

Nevada Association for the Handicapped (NAH)

6200 West Oakey Boulevard
Las Vegas, NV 89146
(702) 870-7050

Services all ages and all types of disabilities. Offers respite care, assisted care, some adult developmental and prevocational training, and some employment services—assessment, training, and placement.

Nevada Association of Latin Americans, Inc.—Arturo Cambeiro Senior Center

330 North Thirteenth Street
Las Vegas, NV 89101
(702) 384-3746

Offers assisted care, some financial assistance, and emergency food assistance.

Nevada Association of Manufactured Home Owners, Inc.

1121 Palm Street

Las Vegas, NV 89104

(702) 384-8428

Educates and informs mobile home owners, offers referrals and some volunteer opportunities, and monitors city, county, and state agencies.

Nevada Caregiver Support Center (NCSC)

(775) 784-4335

www.unr.edu/Sanford/ncsc

Provides education and practical solutions to families and professionals caring for older adults with dementia.

Nevada Council on Problem Gambling

5552 South Fort Apache Road, Suite 100

Las Vegas, NV 89148

(702) 369-9740

Gambling Hotline: (800) 522-4700

Offers telephone reassurance and a referral service.

No to Abuse (NTA)

621 South Blagg Road

Pahrump, NV 89048

(775) 751-1118

Toll Free: (888) 882-2873

http://notoabuse.org

Committed to stopping abuse in the family environment, including elder abuse, child abuse, family violence, and sexual abuse. Offers educational classes in parenting, communications, and crisis intervention training; emergency food assistance; safe shelter; counseling services; and advocacy.

Senior Tripsters, Inc.
451 East Bonanza Road
Las Vegas, NV 89101
(702) 387-0007
    Plans trips for seniors that are as low cost as possible.

Starkey Hearing Foundation—Hear Now
6700 Washington Avenue South
Eden Prairie, MN 55344
Toll Free: (866) 354-3254
    Provides hearing aids to low-income individuals who meet the financial eligibility guidelines.

Supporting Your Journey
Center for Cognitive Aging, University of Nevada School of Medicine
890 Mill Street, Suite 303
Reno, NV 89502
(775) 322-2731
    Support group for those caring for patients in early stages of Alzheimer's disease.

United Way of Northern Nevada
639 Isbell Road
Suite 460
Reno, NV 89509
(775) 332-8668

United Way of Southern Nevada
5830 West Flamingo Road
Las Vegas, NV 89103
(702) 892-2300
    Gives people the opportunity to make a meaningful difference in the lives of others and in the community.

Walter L. Schwartz Center for Compassionate Care

4131 Swenson Street

Las Vegas, NV 89119

(702) 796-3167

Provides services to persons and families in need of information, counseling, consultation, training, and other supportive services.

Government Offices

Nevada Department of Health and Human Services—Welfare District Offices

Belrose District Office

700 Belrose Street

Las Vegas, NV 89107

(702) 486-1646

Cambridge Center

3900 Cambridge Street, Suite 202

Las Vegas, NV 89119

(702) 486-9400

Cannon Center

3330 Flamingo Road, Suite 55

Las Vegas, NV 89121

(702) 486-9400

Carson City District Office

2533 North Carson Street, Suite 200

Carson City, NV 89706

(775) 684-0800

Carson City Energy Assistance Program

2527 North Carson Street, Suite 260

Carson City, NV 89706

(775) 684-0730

Community Assistance Center
1504 North Main Street
Las Vegas, NV 89101
(702) 486-5000

Elko/Winnemucca District Office
1020 Ruby Vista Drive, Suite 101
Elko, NV 89801
(775) 753-1233

Ely District Office
725 Avenue K
Ely, NV 89301
(775) 289-1650

Fallon District Office
111 Industrial Way
Fallon, NV 89406
(775) 423-3161

Flamingo District Office
3330 Flamingo Road, Suite 55
Las Vegas, NV 89121
(702) 486-9400
Senior Services: (702) 486-9500

Hawthorne District Office
1000 C Street
P.O. Box 1508
Hawthorne, NV 89415
(775) 945-3602

Hearings Office and SPDC Quality Control
628 Belrose Street
Las Vegas, NV89107
(702) 486-1437

Henderson District Office

520 South Boulder Highway

Henderson, NV 89015

(702) 486-1001

Nellis District Office

611 North Nellis Boulevard

Las Vegas, NV 89110

(702) 486-4828

Owens District Office

1040 West Owens Avenue

Las Vegas, NV 89106

(702) 486-1899

Pahrump District Office

1840 Pahrump Valley Road

Pahrump, NV 89048

(775) 751-7400

Professional Development Center (North)

680–690 Rock Boulevard

Reno, NV 89502

(775) 448-5240

Professional Development Center (South)

701 North Rancho Drive

Las Vegas, NV 89106

(702) 486-1429

Reno District Office

3697 Kings Row, Suite D

Reno, NV 89503

(775) 684-7200

Southern Nevada Investigations and Recovery Unit

628 Belrose Street

Las Vegas, NV 89107

(702) 486-1875

Winnemucca District Office

3140 Traders Way

Winnemucca, NV 89466

(775) 623-6557

Yerington District Office

215 Bridge Street, Suite 6

Yerington, NV 89447

(775) 463-3028

Nevada Division of Insurance

2501 East Sahara Avenue, Room 302

Las Vegas, NV 89104

(702) 486-4009

1818 East College Parkway, Suite 103

Carson City, NV 89706

(775) 687-0700

Social Security Administration

Toll Free: (800) 772-1213

www.ssa.gov

Assists individuals applying for SSA/SSI benefits and continuing eligibility to such benefits. Answers general questions about Social Security matters.

U.S. Department of Housing and Urban Development

302 East Carson Avenue, Suite 400

Las Vegas, NV 89101

(702) 366-2100

Federal agency with mission of providing a decent, safe, and sanitary home and suitable living environment for every American.

Veterans Services

Department of Veterans Affairs—Reno Regional Office
5460 Reno Corporate Drive
Reno, NV 89511

Mike O'Callaghan Federal Hospital
4700 North Las Vegas Boulevard
Nellis AFB, NV 89191
(702) 653-2273

Nevada State Veterans Nursing Home
100 Veterans Memorial Drive
Boulder City, NV 89005
(702) 332-6864

State-owned facility providing skilled nursing services to veterans, their spouses, and Gold Star parents.

Northern Nevada Veterans Memorial Cemetery
14 Veterans Way
Fernley, NV 89408
(775) 575-4441

North Las Vegas VA Medical Center
6900 North Pecos Road
North Las Vegas NV 89086
(702) 791-9000
www.lasvegas.va.gov

Provides health services for veterans in Southern Nevada, including specialty care, surgery, mental health services, and rehabilitation and support programs.

Reno Veterans Administration Medical Center—Geriatric and Extended-Care Program
1000 Locust Street
Reno, NV 89502
(775) 786-7200

Southern Nevada Veterans Memorial Cemetery
1900 Veterans Memorial Drive
Boulder City, NV 89005
(702) 486-5920

Veterans Administration General Information
Toll Free: (800) 827-1000

Veterans Administration Regional Office
5460 Reno Corporate Drive
Reno, NV 89511
Toll Free: (800) 827-1000

Veterans Assistance Office (Northern Nevada)
1155 West 4th Street, Suite 101
Reno, NV 89503
(775) 323-1294

Veterans Assistance Office (Southern Nevada)
1919 South Jones Boulevard
Las Vegas, NV 89146
(702) 251-7873

Web Sites and Useful Telephone Numbers

American Academy of Neurology
www.aan.com
   Provides a list of neurologists.

Benefits Checkup

www.benefitscheckup.org

For people age fifty-five or older who may need programs to assist them with prescription drugs, health care, utilities, and other items or services.

Innovaging

www.innovaging.com

A resource guide for seniors in the Carson City and Reno-Sparks areas.

Living Will Lockbox

www.livingwilllockbox.com

A virtual, secure lockbox for filing living wills and other documents for easy access by medical providers.

Medicare

www.medicare.gov

Provides more information on Medicare.

National Academy of Elder Law Attorneys

(520) 881-4005

www.naela.org

Provides a list of certified elder law attorneys.

National Association of Professional Geriatric Care Managers

www.caremanager.org

Provides a list of geriatric care managers.

National Do Not Call Registry

Toll Free: (888) 382-1222

www.donotcall.gov

If you register with the Do Not Call Registry, you will substantially limit the number of telemarketing calls you receive.

Nevada-2-1-1

http://nevada211.org

Call Nevada 2-1-1 for any basic need, health, or human service program.

Nevada Care Connection

http://www.nevadaadrc.com

Provides resources for Nevada caregivers.

Nevada Health Link

www.nevadahealthlink.com

The online marketplace created by the State of Nevada where individuals and businesses can shop for health insurance plans.

Reporting Scams

Call the state attorney general at (800) 266-8688 or (775) 486-3777. You can also contact the National Fraud Information Center at (800) 876-7060.

SeniorNet Web

www.seniornet.org

Provides nonprofit computer and Internet education for seniors.

Bottke, Allison. *Setting Boundaries With Your Aging Parents.* Eugene, OR: Harvest House Publishers, 2010.

Brody, Elaine M. *Women in the Middle: Their Parent-Care Years.* 2d ed. New York: Spring Press, 2003.

Collier, Victoria. *47 Secret Veterans' Benefits for Seniors.* Scottdale, GA: Collier Communications, 2010.

Delehanty, Hugh. *Caring for Your Parents: The Complete Family Guide.* New York, NY: Sterling Publishing, 2008.

Doka, Kenneth J., ed. *Improving Care for Veterans Facing Illness and Death.* Washington, DC: Hospice Foundation of America, 2013.

———. *Living with Grief: Alzheimer's Disease.* Washington, DC: Hospice Foundation of America, 2004.

———. *Living with Grief After Sudden Loss.* Washington, DC: Hospice Foundation of America, 1996.

Graboys, Thomas, with Peter Zheutlin. *Life in the Balance: A Physician's Memoir of Life, Love, and Loss with Parkinson's Disease and Dementia.* New York/London: Union Square Press, 2008.

Haber, David. *Health Promotion and Aging: Practical Applications for Health Professionals.* 6th ed. New York: Springer Publishing, 2013.

Kassai, Kathryn, and Perelli, Kim. *The Bathroom Key: Put an End to Incontinence.* New York: Demos Medical Publishing, 2011.

Lane, Kathy. *Die Smart: 11 Mistakes That Cost Your Family When You Die: Probate, Living Trusts, Power of Attorney (and More).* Half Moon Bay, CA: NFormed, 2011.

Lindbergh, Reeve. *No More Words: A Journal of My Mother, Anne Morrow Lindbergh.* New York: Simon & Schuster, 2002.

Mace, Nancy L., and Peter V. Rabins. *The 36-Hour Day.* Baltimore, MD: Warner Books, by special agreement with the Johns Hopkins University Press, 1992.

Margolies, Linda. *My Mother's Hip: Lessons from the World of Eldercare.* Philadelphia, PA: Temple University Press, 2004.

Markut, Lynda, and Anatole Crane. *Dementia Caregivers Share Their Stories: A Support Group in a Book.* Nashville, TN: Vanderbilt University Press, 2005.

Roche, John. *The Veteran's Survival Guide: How to File and Collect on VA Claims.* 2d ed. Dulles, VA: Potomac Books, 2006.

Senelick, Richard C. *Living with Stroke: A Guide for Families.* Ashland, OH: Healthsouth Press, 2010.

Strong, Maggie. *Mainstay: For the Well Spouse of the Chronically Ill.* Northhampton, MA: Bardford Books, 1998.

Tate, Nick J. *ObamaCare Survival Guide.* West Palm Beach, FL: Humanix Books, 2013.

Vad, Vijay. *Arthritis Rx: A Cutting-Edge Program for a Pain-Free Life.* New York: Gotham, 2007.

INDEX

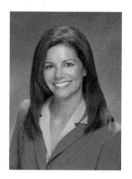

Kim Boyer is a certified elder law attorney and founder of Boyer Law Group, where she practices in the areas of elder law, guardianship, probate, Medicaid and veterans' benefits, and long-term care planning. She is a frequent speaker on aging and elder law topics and was named as one of the Top 40 Women Attorneys in the Mountain States area.

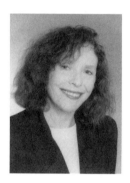

Mary Shapiro is a gerontologist, geriatric care manager, and cofounder of Senior Direction, LLC, a geriatric care management company. Ms. Shapiro facilitates support groups for those dealing with Parkinson's disease, dementia, and Alzheimer's disease. She presents ongoing workshops on aging, Alzheimer's, and dementia for professionals and the general public.

In addition to this book, Kim Boyer and Mary Shapiro are co-authors of the book *Alzheimer's and Dementia: A Practical and Legal Guide for Nevada Caregivers,* published by the University of Nevada Press. Both authors live and work in Las Vegas. You can learn more by visiting their websites www.elderlawnv.com and www.seniordirection.net.